HEARING VOICES

HEARING VOICES
QUALITATIVE INQUIRY IN EARLY PSYCHOSIS

Katherine M. Boydell and H. Bruce Ferguson, editors

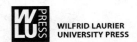

WILFRID LAURIER UNIVERSITY PRESS

SickKids®

Wilfrid Laurier University Press acknowledges the financial support of the Government of Canada through the Canada Book Fund for our publishing activities.

Library and Archives Canada Cataloguing in Publication

Hearing voices : qualitative inquiry in early psychosis / Katherine M. Boydell and H. Bruce Ferguson, editors.

(SickKids community and mental health series)
Includes bibliographical references and index.
Also issued in electronic format.
ISBN 978-1-55458-263-1

1. Psychoses. 2. Psychoses—Treatment. I. Boydell, Katherine II. Ferguson, H. Bruce III. Series: SickKids community and mental health series

RC512.H42 2012   616.89   C2011-907608-X

Electronic monograph.
Also issued in print format.
ISBN 978-1-55458-310-2 (PDF). — ISBN 978-1-55458-885-5 (EPUB)

1. Psychoses. 2. Psychoses—Treatment. I. Boydell, Katherine II. Ferguson, H. Bruce III. Series: SickKids community and mental health series (Online)

RC512.H42 2012   616.89   C2011-907609-8

Cover design by Chris Rowat Design. Front-cover image: *Breaking Free* (acrylic paint), by Roberto Louis Foz. Text design by Daiva Villa, Chris Rowat Design.

This book is printed on FSC recycled paper and is certified Ecologo. It is made from 100% post-consumer fibre, processed chlorine free, and manufactured using biogas energy.

Printed in Canada

Published by Wilfrid Laurier University Press
Waterloo, Ontario, Canada
www.wlupress.wlu.ca

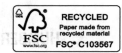

Contents

Preface

Katherine M. Boydell

In Canada and internationally, recent years have witnessed an increased growth in qualitative inquiry in the health sciences. Qualitative research exploring the social determinants of health, clinical decision making, interaction between practitioners and patients, patient experiences of illness, health care delivery, and other social aspects of health and health care are regularly featured in medical, nursing, and other health research and professional journals. This text is based on an international symposium featuring such qualitative inquiry in the field of early psychosis, which was held in Toronto in October 2007. Research in the field of early psychosis needs to draw on different perspectives, methodologies, and techniques to generate breadth of knowledge and depth of understanding. Qualitative research is a broad umbrella term for research methodologies that describe and explain individual experiences, behaviours, interactions, and social contexts without the use of statistical procedures or quantification. The aim of most forms of qualitative research is to understand how the world is socially constructed by its participants as well as what meanings those constructions have for the participants. Qualitative methodologies are particularly appropriate for understanding individuals' and groups' subjective experiences of health and disease; social, cultural, and political factors in health and disease; and interactions among participants within health care settings.

Qualitative research questions focus chiefly on three areas: (1) language as a means to explore processes of communication and patterns of interaction within particular social groups; (2) the description and interpretation of subjective meanings attributed to situations and actions; and (3) theory building through discovering patterns and connections in the data. These methodologies have much to offer in the field of early intervention. This volume highlights the research that has been conducted internationally and illustrates its' potential for impact at both the levels of service delivery and mental health policy.

The first half of the book is structured around the individual lived experience of psychosis—from the individual, family, and practitioner's perspectives. The second half moves the reader beyond the micro level towards the macro level, focusing on broader system issues such as medical trainees' encounters with first episode psychosis (FEP) in the emergency room and the implementation of first episode clinics in the United Kingdom and Australia.

Jean Addington begins with an overview of the current state of empirical knowledge on early intervention. She affirms that the clinical and research practice in FEP accomplished to date constitutes a major reform in the treatment of schizophrenia. Tremendous shifts have been made worldwide to identify and treat young people at the very beginning of their illness. Programs have been, and are continuing to be, developed worldwide. The FEP field expects that treatments for people newly diagnosed with a psychotic illness should be available right at the beginning of their illness and that such treatments will need to be of the highest quality and aimed at the best recovery possible. She calls on researchers to further understand the ways in which mental illness interferes with everyday life and how people can learn to manage and minimize the illness so that they can pursue their lives to the best of their ability even in the face of persisting illness. Qualitative methods are uniquely well suited to this task.

Katherine Boydell and her colleagues present early findings from their series of case studies focusing on the pathways to mental health care. They highlight a particular case to illustrate the role of illness recognition and (mis)attribution, the experience of symptoms as reality, and the need for education and awareness in the pathway to mental health care. Identification of the various facilitators and roadblocks in accessing services will contribute to our understanding of the duration of untreated psychosis. By taking a comprehensive approach to understanding this journey, the dynamic complexity and interrelatedness of the role of the family, school, treatment system, and broader community are revealed.

Katherine Boydell, Siona Jackson, and John Strauss describe a research-based dance production that aims to provide knowledge about first episode psychosis in an accessible and meaningful way to a wide variety of audiences. The linking of qualitative research to artistic productions is a new and innovative field that has enormous potential to make research more vital, tangible, and relevant. Empirical qualitative data on the subjective, everyday experience of help seeking, as described by ten young people between the ages of sixteen and twenty-four, was expressed using movement and music (the dance). The performance presents the responses of young people to the first signs of psychosis, the factors that motivated their response, and the role that others played in help seeking. It highlights both the particularity and the universality of their stories.

Ruth Gerson and Cheryl Corcoran note that qualitative research with families is important for understanding the behavioural manifestations in the early stages of psychotic disorders and for discerning what is helpful to these young individuals and their families. They describe findings from qualitative interviews with family members of young people who are experiencing the recent onset of non-affective psychosis. A striking theme in the narratives is the profound suffering that these families and patients are experiencing. The families are grappling for meaning and understanding, and their attributions of symptoms include stress, drug use, spiritual crisis, normal adolescence, and genetic risk for mental illness. They describe not knowing what to do, feeling "tired" and "helpless, like pounding on a brick wall." They report difficulties navigating the health care system and the feeling of a considerable sense of burden. Clearly, these young people and their families deserve early, accessible, and affordable services, which may not only prevent or forestall the onset of psychosis but also address the significant decline in social and role function that has been observed.

Helen Lester explores the potential roles and responsibilities of the primary care team in providing care and advice for people with FEP. Primary care practitioners require easy access to specialist advice and assessment skills for individuals with suspected FEP, who could then be referred to less stigmatizing and more easily accessible environments. Early intervention services also have a role to play in addressing the knowledge gaps experienced by general practitioners and their attitudes towards young people with FEP. When such levels of partnership between primary care and early intervention clinics working are achieved, care pathways may become less time consuming to manoeuvre and less traumatic.

There is very little in the existing literature that examines the lessons that doctors have learned from their ordinary and extraordinary interactions with patients—experience that is referred to as the hidden curriculum of learning. What can we learn about an individual with early stage psychosis if we view the experience from the perspective of clinicians who care for these people? Joan McIlwrick draws on qualitative data from experienced clinicians as well as on the reflections of more novice residents regarding individuals with early psychosis. Results indicate that the patient's experience is the constant teacher and that the clinician must be a lifelong student. No matter how many years of experience the veteran interventionist develops, McIlwrick's data suggest that in the case of early psychosis the lessons they have learned can be the same as those learned by the novice early interventionist. This realization is critical for all early interventionists to remember due to the increasing expectations from both public and private international organizations, looking to determine measurable outcomes from early intervention teams.

Studies of the impact of staff reorientation and retraining are still a relative rarity in the early psychosis field, and it is essential that we understand their implications so that we can improve and sustain such re-skilling processes and outcomes. Alan Rosen and his colleagues address this extant gap through their examination of clinician attitudes towards early psychosis intervention programs and the impact of change strategies on staff attitudes. Their study utilizes both diffusion theory and concerns theory to develop a questionnaire that explores staff attitudes as well as examines and facilitates the process of change. Most of their respondents indicated that they expected early intervention to provide better outcomes for clients and families, although they did not necessarily think it would be more cost-effective or beneficial for staff. Respondents were undecided about their own readiness to provide early psychosis intervention, and they suggested that some of the barriers to implementation included a lack of knowledge or skills rather than an unfavourable attitude. Concerns were expressed about resources, particularly about resources that might have been allocated to this innovation at the expense of longer-term clients. Dissemination strategies, such as the use of educational programs and restructuring services, that were developed during the thirty-six-month study period resulted in a positive shift in staff attitudes towards early intervention. Evidence of management's support for such innovation, particularly service restructuring, at Time 1 and the employment of a project officer after Time 2 are factors that are likely to have contributed to the resolution of personal concerns by Time 3.

Sue Estroff reflects on interventions for first episode and early psychosis and considers whether and how qualitative inquiry can inform and influence clinical and research approaches to early intervention in psychosis. She casts both a skeptical and a hopeful gaze on how research using qualitative methods provides evidence of the risks and rewards of interventions for people whose experiences with psychosis and treatment are emergent, recent, and unfamiliar. This chapter is timely as the proliferation of early psychosis clinics across the world demands that we inquire as to the subjective experience of those people impacted by psychosis and the social contexts within which it occurs and is lived out.

The chapters in this text include international research, which makes use of qualitative inquiry to explore processes of communication and patterns of interaction; to describe and interpret subjective meanings; and to use and build theory. The individual lived experience of psychosis is explored from the individual, family, and practitioner's perspectives. Moving from the individual level to the systemic level, chapters highlight medical trainees' encounters with FEP in the emergency room and the implementation of first episode clinics in the United Kingdom and Australia.

Acknowledgements

I would like to extend my sincere thanks to Bruce Ferguson for his constant support and encouragement and his unwavering commitment to developing community capacity to improve outcomes for children and youth.

I am indebted to Sarah Bovaird for her role in planning the symposium upon which this text is based and to Karima Kinlock for her coordination of the people and materials needed in order to make this book a reality. It has been a privilege to work with such an amazing group of researchers and clinicians who contributed book chapters that demonstrate their commitment to study early psychosis qualitatively.

I owe my deepest gratitude to my research team—Brenda, Elaine, and Tiz. Your contributions to all we do are appreciated and you make work on every research project a pleasurable experience.

To my husband David and daughters Cristina, Alexandra, and Ariana: your love is a constant in my life.

This book was made possible through financial support from The Hospital for Sick Children and from The Canadian Institutes of Health Research

Katherine Boydell

I want to thank the authors of this volume for bringing breadth and intensity to this important area. I am grateful to my co-editors for creating a process that was always committed to excellence but also edifying and fun. Sarah Bovaird and Karima Kinlock worked hard to make it easy for me to contribute to the process. Finally, I would like to acknowledge the members of the Community Health Systems Resource Group at SickKids, whose passion, focus, and knowledge keep me humble and curious and maintain my conviction that together we can and will make a difference in the lives of our children and youth.

H. Bruce Ferguson

Abbreviations

ARMS	at-risk mental states
CBT	cognitive behavioural therapy
CMHTs	community mental health teams
DUP	duration of untreated psychosis
EIS	early intervention services
EPI	early psychosis intervention
EPPIC	Early Psychosis Prevention and Intervention Clinic
EPPINY	Early Psychosis Prevention and Intervention Network for Young People
FEP	first episode psychosis
GP	general practitioner
IEPA	International Early Psychosis Association
NEM	Network Episode Model
NIMH	National Institute of Mental Health
RCTs	randomized controlled trials
RCT	randomized controlled trial

Introduction to Early Intervention in First Episode Psychosis

Jean Addington

Interest in first episode psychosis (FEP) and its early intervention began almost twenty years ago. It is now a rapidly expanding field that is part of the mainstream of psychiatry and mental health. Early intervention for psychosis is actually a growth point within the schizophrenia field with exponential development in basic research, clinical research, clinical care, and health services research. There are some key landmarks that have marked the beginning of this movement of research, education, treatment, and advocacy. In the 1990s, many individuals became increasingly optimistic about the possibility of improved outcomes for individuals with schizophrenia and other psychoses due to several findings, including, first, evidence of the impact of a long duration of untreated psychosis (DUP); second, the benefits of intervening early for subsequent recovery; third, the notion that the first three to five years following the illness onset is a critical period for intervention; and, finally, the advent of the second generation of antipsychotics.

The work of the Australian group at the University of Melbourne led by Patrick McGorry has had an unparalleled impact on the field. Concerned with the quality of routine traditional clinical care for schizophrenia patients, the delay in receiving such treatment for those suffering from a FEP, and the fact that most people do not have access to potentially effective pharmacological and psychosocial treatments, this group set up the Early Psychosis Prevention and Intervention Clinic (EPPIC). EPPIC has become one of the most comprehensive innovative programs dedicated to the treatment of those individuals experiencing a FEP.

Interestingly, this focus on early intervention could be viewed not as a demand for "early intervention" but, rather, as an "on-time intervention" as these young people could already have been diagnosed with schizophrenia or other psychotic disorders. Thus, the first stage of this "early intervention" movement was to offer as soon as possible a wide range of treatments that were appropriate to the stage of the illness and to the age of those with the disorder. It also served to address psychosis in all of its forms as early and as intensely as possible. Today, early intervention is a movement that has spread worldwide. Programs and services have, and continue to be, developed throughout the world. There exists an international organization known as the International Early Psychosis Association, which has over 2,500 members representing more than sixty countries. Recently, a journal representing an interest in early intervention in psychiatry—*Early Intervention in Psychiatry*—was launched. Work in early intervention and early psychosis has grown to include those individuals who are clinically at high risk of developing a psychotic illness—that is, those who are presenting with attenuated psychotic symptoms who could potentially be prodromal for psychosis.

In comparison to "standard care," early intervention for a FEP aims to identify as soon as possible people who are already psychotic but who have not yet received adequate treatment. This effort is then followed by phase-specific treatments with the intention of promoting recovery from a FEP. Specialized treatment can occur in programs already offering "standard care," or it can be obtained through specialized early intervention teams. Early intervention services typically offer a range of interventions enriched specifically to address issues relevant to this early phase of the illness and particular group of patients. Delivery of care can be flexible and is often based on a case management program. These programs have been termed "multi-element" programs since they offer a comprehensive array of specialized in- and out-patient services emphasizing both symptomatic and functional recovery. Many of the problems for young individuals experiencing psychosis, such as substance abuse, suicidality, and engagement in the health system, are addressed through a range of targeted therapeutic approaches.

A large number of early psychosis clinical and research programs have been established worldwide, and in the last decade these newly established clinical and research programs have developed into large-scale networks of programs with interest groups, diverse service initiatives, and national and international conferences throughout many countries and regions, including, for example, Australia, Canada, the United Kingdom, Switzerland, the Netherlands, Scandinavia, Germany, Singapore, and Hong Kong. There is an ever-increasing body of literature on program development, and resources are readily available for a variety of initiatives. Although there are no clear "standards of care" yet developed, numerous clinical guidelines for FEP have been published (International Early Psychosis Association [IEPA] Writing Group, 2005).

There is a wide range of studies examining FEP (see Addington, 2007). Some are cross-sectional and are essentially descriptive of this population, while others are longitudinal and report on changes over time. Some of them are real world effectiveness studies. Some studies evaluate multi-element interventions, which typically include community outreach, early detection efforts, in- and out-patient treatment, individual, group, and family treatment, case management, and pharmacological treatment, or others evaluate specific single-element psychosocial interventions (for example, cognitive behaviour therapy [CBT] or a medication approach). Treatment outcome studies tend to be uncontrolled, although a few use a historical control group, and randomized clinical trials are rare.

By examining certain constructs at the beginning of schizophrenia or other psychotic illnesses, we have learned that individuals at the first episode often show compromised cognitive functioning, with deficits that are often comparable to those with a more chronic course of illness. Furthermore, these young patients have impaired social functioning, and, unfortunately, functional recovery does not match symptomatic recovery. Another often-studied variable is the period or DUP because, unlike other prognostic factors, it has the potential to be reduced through changes in health service delivery. An understanding of the pathways to care—that is, an awareness of the number of attempts an individual has made to obtain help and who is the most likely to ensure appropriate treatment is obtained—is a prerequisite for early detection and the effective treatment of FEP. This research reveals certain common themes: pathways to care are highly varied and diverse; health professionals are usually first contact; there is considerable delay in treatment, irrespective of the setting; some delay occurs because of the failure of caregivers and primary care in recognizing incipient psychosis; and there is a delay in initiating treatment for psychosis in those who are already engaged in mental health services.

Randomized controlled trials (RCTs) determining the impact of FEP treatment are rare, but they offer preliminary support for the advantages of early intervention. In support, a wide range of well-described and well-established FEP programs are reporting improved symptomatic and functional outcomes in comparison to historical control groups, while others that are epidemiologically representative are also reporting positive outcomes. Good intermediate outcome is more common. There are also studies that are beginning to examine the impact of single elements in programs such as family intervention, CBT, pharmacology, and substance use treatment. Issues such as relapse, suicide, and substance use are also being explored.

The clinical and research practice in FEP that has been accomplished to date constitutes a major reform in the treatment of schizophrenia. Tremendous shifts have been made worldwide to identify and treat young people at the very beginning of their illness. Programs have been, and are continuing to be, developed worldwide. The FEP field expects that treatments for people newly diagnosed with a psychotic illness should be available right at the beginning of the illness and that such treatment needs to be of the highest quality and aimed at the best recovery possible.

Typically, criticisms of early intervention reflect the notion that although it is a well-established approach in many countries it is unclear how much early detection, phase-specific treatments, and early intervention teams are supported by evidence of effectiveness. A recent review has demonstrated that there are successful reports of reduction in DUP (Addington, 2007). Pathways to care are being explored with the intent of better understanding and subsequently improving referral systems. Traditionally, outcome in schizophrenia has had a major focus on psychopathology. However, increasingly, occupational and social functioning as well as the person's quality of life are being seen as even more important measurements of the impact of the illness and/or its treatment. Once we have made a diagnosis, we now have concerns about how these young people will adapt to the illness and what the impact will be on their development, and, thus, we are striving to lessen this impact. Substance use, medication side effects, and relapse rates are being studied and addressed. Successful work with families to help them deal with their distress is also being reported. RCTs are rare, but effectiveness studies are highly promising. We have a range of evidence of improved adherence and decreased attrition, of a reduction in positive and negative symptoms, and of a reduction in depression, hopelessness, suicide, and relapse rates.

We have to date made good progress. However, the potential for improving the outcome of patients through earlier intervention is likely to be limited unless it is combined with improved treatment that is specifically designed for this early first phase of illness and for a younger patient population. We do need to ensure that FEP programs are properly implemented. We need to make use of available performance measures for early psychosis treatment services to establish standards and norms for routine clinical practice. Intervention at the FEP is a complex intervention of early engagement, maintaining engagement, reducing DUP, and offering well-developed, phase-specific interventions.

In research, future work needs to focus on an improved understanding of the delay in treatment both from the "seeking" perspective of the client, the referral perspective of gatekeepers, and the delivery of treatment. We need to pay attention to cultural, social, and political issues. In addition, there has to be longer-term data from large cohorts of FEP patients that includes uniform assessment procedures and clearly defined multi-dimensional criteria for determining a patient's outcome. Large epidemiologically representative samples are required with a minimum of two to three year follow-up interviews. Non-adherence with treatment and relapse rates are crucial issues. The impact of treatments needs to be monitored for quality of delivery and effectiveness. Many more RCTs are needed in order to determine not just if a treatment is effective but also for whom it may be effective and at what stage of the recovery process it will have the most impact. We have to find ways to understand the different trajectories of outcome so that we can better define the patient subgroups that follow the different trajectories.

There remains uncertainty about the length of time for which treatment should continue and what the follow-up procedure should look like beyond the FEP program. A legitimate concern is that the FEP program may be offering an intensive treatment that will no longer be available for patients after they are discharged from the program. It also remains questionable whether early intervention programs can offer the prospect of altering the course of schizophrenia without a sustained comprehensive treatment program.

Without a doubt, there is an active and dedicated network of clinicians and researchers working in early psychosis who are interested in sharing information, resources, and data to ensure the future of service developments. To further inform this community and to accelerate such progress, our research efforts not only need to be of the highest quality, but they also have to continue to be accompanied by political pressure and community demand.

This volume focuses on the recognition that qualitative methods are becoming increasingly useful as psychiatry shifts away from symptom reduction and moves towards enabling people to live satisfying, hopeful, and meaningful lives in the community (Davidson, Ridgway, Kidd, Topor, and Borg, 2008). Consequently, it is becoming essential that researchers further understand the ways in which mental illness interferes with everyday life and the ways in which people can learn to manage and minimize the illness so that they can pursue their lives to the best of their abilities even in the face of persisting illness. Qualitative methods are uniquely well suited for this task. Qualitative research is not new to psychiatry, as is evidenced by such classical textbooks as Erving Goffman's *Asylums* (1963) and William Caudill's *The Psychiatric Hospital as a Small Society* (1958), which use ethnographic methods of participant observation. These methods were introduced to community psychiatry by Sue Estroff (1981) in her landmark text *Making It Crazy*. A special edition of the *Schizophrenia Bulletin* in 1989, co-edited by John Strauss and Estroff (1989), highlights the need to use qualitative methods to examine the lived experience of individuals with serious and persistent mental illness. Since its publication, there has been a burgeoning of qualitative inquiry in the mental health field. Although there has been a dramatic surge in the literature using qualitative methods in psychiatry in general, only a handful of studies have been published that use such methods specifically to explore the lives, both socio-culturally and experientially, of young people with FEP (see recent review by Boydell, Stasiulis, Volpe, and Gladstone, 2010).

Historically, most outcome studies in FEP have tended to adopt quantitative methods and have focused on a biomedical model, using standardized measures of symptomatology, social functioning, and quality of life. What has been missing in this work is the importance of exploring the subjective experience of individuals experiencing psychosis as well as the significance of listening to the person's story about his or her life and illness experiences. For example, we know that a lack of compliance with medication and dropping out of treatment are common issues in first episode clinics; however, we lack understanding of the circumstances and contexts in which these decisions are made. Qualitative inquiry can assist in this undertaking as we seek to ask, listen to, and learn from these individuals. Clearly, research in the field needs to draw on different perspectives, methodologies, and techniques to generate a breadth of knowledge and a depth of understanding. The chapters in this volume highlight the lived experience of young people with FEP, their families, and the health care practitioners.

References

Addington, J. (2007). The promise of early intervention. *Journal of Early Intervention, 1*, 294-307.

Boydell, K.M., Stasiulis, E., Volpe, T., and Gladstone, B.M. (2010). A descriptive review of qualitative inquiry in early psychosis. *Early Intervention in Psychiatry, 4*, 7-24.

Caudill, W. (1958). *The psychiatric hospital as a small society*. Boston, MA: Harvard University Press.

Davidson, L., Ridgway, P., Kidd, S., Topor, A., and Borg, M. (2008). Using qualitative research to inform mental health policy. *Canadian Journal of Psychiatry, 53*(3), 137-44.

Estroff, S.E. (1981). *Making it crazy: An ethnography of psychiatric clients in an American community.* Berkeley, CA: University of California Press.

Goffman, E. (1963). *Stigma: Notes on the management of spoiled identity.* New York, NY: Simon and Schuster.

International Early Psychosis Association (IEPA) Writing Group. (2005). International clinical practice guidelines for early psychosis (supplemental material). *British Journal of Psychiatry, 48*, 120-24.

Strauss, J.S., and Estroff, S.E. (1989). Introduction to the special issue. *Schizophrenia Bulletin, 15*(2), 177-78.

1

Recognition of Psychosis in the Pathway to Mental Health Care

Katherine M. Boydell, Elaine Stasiulis, Brenda M. Gladstone,
Tiziana Volpe, Jean Addington, Paula Goering, Terry Krupa,
and Elizabeth McCay

Introduction

In the field of psychiatry, detection and intervention in the early stages of schizophrenia offer hope for substantial improvements in schizophrenia and schizophrenia spectrum disorders (Addington, 2007). Studies indicate that 2 percent of adolescents in Canada experience psychosis, which is often a precursor to schizophrenia (McMaster University, 2003). Psychosis is described as a disorganization of thoughts and emotional responses and the inability to recognize reality (Lines, 2000). Common symptoms include significant changes in behaviour, social isolation, feelings of suspicion, unusual beliefs, hearing voices, seeing things, and mood changes. The process of becoming psychotic creates profound psychological changes that are frightening, difficult to comprehend, and isolating. The consequent disruption of social networks, including family and peer relationships, as well as of schoolwork and occupational functioning, can be devastating (Addington, Leriger, and Addington, 2003; Addington, Young, and Addington, 2003). First episode psychosis (FEP) has been identified as a "critical period" for intervention to prevent further impairments and the best time to instigate bio-psychosocial interventions. However, many youth with psychosis do not appear to seek help. Their family and friends fail to comprehend the enormity of the changes occurring, and their psychosis is often overlooked or misdiagnosed. As a result, there are significant delays between the onset of symptoms and the initiation of treatment. This duration of untreated psychosis (DUP) is critical, given the evidence suggesting a strong relationship between the length of untreated psychosis and poor clinical and social outcomes (Addington, van Mastrigt, Hutchinson, and Addington, 2002). Consequently, it is important to know the extant barriers and facilitators in the pathway to accessing mental health care.

Background

Our current understanding of help seeking by youth with psychiatric problems in general and with psychosis in particular is limited. Yet understanding how the various services and supports are obtained in the early stages of psychosis is critical for early intervention (Lincoln and McGorry, 1995). Worldwide studies have revealed that individuals suffering from a FEP experience an alarming delay between the onset of psychotic symptoms and the initiation of treatment (Addington, van Mastrigt, and Addington, 2004; Lieberman and Fenton, 2000; Malla, Norman, McLean, Scholten, and Townsend, 2003; Norman and Malla, 2001). Examining the factors that contribute to this delay is essential, as early psychiatric intervention not only significantly aids recovery in FEP but may also reduce subsequent chronic symptomatology (Birchwood, 1992; Birchwood, and Macmillan, 1993; Falloon, 1992). Furthermore, understanding the help-seeking process is fundamental to designing more effective service delivery as well as to addressing the needs of the underserved and assisting youth and their significant others in making decisions about seeking mental health intervention (Richardson, 2001). Actively learning from individuals and their significant others will assist service providers and policy makers in planning more efficient pathways to mental health services (Addington et al., 2002).

There is currently no comprehensive theoretical model that addresses methodological and conceptual issues in understanding pathways to treatment for youth with FEP. Such a model should include the involvement of young people and their significant others to ensure that services meet their needs (Lincoln and McGorry, 1995). Christine Lincoln and Patrick McGorry (1995) have suggested that the experiences inherent in the narratives of consumers of care service and their caregivers are fundamental to future research that seeks to understand how pathways are experienced and negotiated (Lincoln and McGorry, 1999). To understand the help-seeking behaviour of young people, one must consider concurrently the various ways in which they come to obtain care, the influence of the various community-based factors, and the impact of circumstances that influence both their modes of entry and their ties to their social network (Ho and Andreasen, 2001; Morgan, Mallett, Hutchinson, and Leff, 2004). This study aims to address this gap in knowledge by using the Network Episode Model (NEM) (Pescosolido, 1992; 1998), which has been adapted for children and youth as a framework to explore the illness career, role of significant others, and the service and support system for youth experiencing FEP (Costello, Pescosolido, Angold, and Burns, 1998).

The NEM reconceptualizes earlier pathway models, systematically considering the varied social processes through which individuals come to enter psychiatric treatment (Aday and Andersen, 1974; Andersen, 1995; Andersen and Newman, 1973). It takes a broad view of individuals with mental health problems and their entry into care and makes no one assumption about how individuals come into treatment. Most importantly, the model illuminates the importance of social influence (enacted through community social networks) on when, how, and whether individuals receive care. The NEM is primarily concerned with the illness career and the process through which individuals enter treatment. It describes and documents processes while simultaneously elaborating on the range and nature of factors that shape an individual's service use. The processes of social influence mediated by contacts in the social network replace the previous isolated and individualistic pathway models that assume that the decision to seek help is an individual one. In other words, people face illness in the course of their day-to-day lives, and in their interactions with others they may be helped to recognize as well as to deny the problems. For instance, others may refer them for treatment or may provide services and support and influence the person along the pathway to care, including something, for example, as simple as reminding them about medical appointments.

Jane Costello and her colleagues (1998) reconceptualized the NEM to underscore the special circumstances of mental health care use for children and youth. In their adaptation, they found that two critical modifications were necessary. First, the family is required to play a more significant role than it might otherwise play in services for adults. Second, the school is viewed as a critical, institutional support system for children. Along with parents, the school is a significant factor in the process of recognizing and managing the mental health issues of children and youth.

The Case Study Approach

A case study approach was used to document the help-seeking pathways of youth experiencing FEP. Case studies involve "an in-depth analysis of a discrete entity (a single setting, subject, collection, or event) on the assumption that it is possible to derive knowledge of a wider phenomenon from an intensive investigation of a specific instance or case" (Yin, 1994, p. 44). By concentrating on a single phenomenon or entity, the goal was to uncover the interaction of significant factors characteristic of that phenomenon or entity. In this study, the single phenomena or unit of analysis was the "pathway to mental health care."

The case study approach involved an in-depth examination of the pathways to mental health care using data from eight index cases.[1] It encompassed thirty-six interviews with youth and significant others—including parents, general practitioners (GPs), friends, guidance counsellors, a psychiatrist, sibling, and vice-principal—involved in the help-seeking process. Purposive, criterion-based selection was used to select the index cases (Patton, 1990). Cases were based on predetermined attributes identified in the literature and in our own clinical and research work. More specifically, this selection strategy provided information-rich cases that varied on key dimensions—for example, length of untreated psychosis, geographic location, ethnicity, gender, substance use, and age (LeCompte and Preissle, 1993).

Inclusion criteria for the index cases included youth aged sixteen to twenty-four years, currently stabilized, and recently enrolled (less than one year) in two FEP programs. Youth were diagnosed according to the criteria set out by the fourth edition of the *Diagnostic and Statistical Manual of Mental Disorders (DSM-IV)* (2000), using the structured clinical interview (SCID-I) (Spitzer, Williams, Gibbons, and First, 1992). Inter-rater reliability was determined by 100 percent agreement on the diagnosis and at least 80 percent agreement for symptom presence. Youth were included if they met one or more of the following schizophrenia spectrum disorders: schizophrenia, schizophreniform disorder, schizoaffective disorder, delusional disorder, brief psychotic disorder, and psychotic disorder not otherwise specified. Youth were willing to identify and consent to contacting the significant others who were involved in their pathway, were English speaking, and were able to consent to participate. Participants were excluded if they were at serious risk of suicide or violence to others or had a primary diagnosis of drug-induced psychosis or psychosis due to a general medical condition.

Cases were recruited from first episode clinics in two Canadian cities. Individuals who indicated an interest in participating were screened to determine suitability, using the SCID-I administered routinely by FEP clinical staff. All individuals who met the criteria for inclusion were asked to provide their consent to be contacted by the research co-ordinator, who subsequently obtained informed consent from those who indicated an interest in participating following a more detailed description of the study.

Basic demographic information was collected for all participants at the outset of each qualitative interview. Two semi-structured interviews were conducted with each participant, and these interviews were approximately twelve weeks apart. Additionally, at the end of the first interview, young people were asked to identify up to four individuals in their formal and informal support network whom they considered to have information related to their pathway to mental health care. The researcher probed for those individuals who helped as well as those who posed barriers to getting help. Following Bernice Pescosolido (1998), one-time interviews with significant others were conducted following the Time 1 interviews with youth. Based on the interviews with youth (Time 1) and significant others, a schematic of the pathway to care was constructed for each case. This schema was then presented to the youth in the second qualitative interview for feedback and discussion. Youth were asked to comment and reflect on their own pathway to care, taking into account the influence of others in their social network (community, family, and school) in the help-seeking process.

Textual data from interviews and field notes were analyzed in three phases, involving: (1) the provision of analysis and description of each case and themes within each case (a within-case analysis); (2) an interpretation of the meaning of the case to allow for a rich elaboration of the context of the case or the setting in which the case presented itself; and (3) a thematic analysis across cases (a cross-case analysis). All interviews were audio-taped and transcribed verbatim. The work of Virginia Braun and Victoria Clarke (2006) informed the coding strategies undertaken in the analysis. First, research team members (Katherine Boydell, Elaine Stasiulis, Brenda Gladstone, Tiziana Volpe) familiarized themselves with the data by reading and rereading each transcript (interviews and field notes). At this point, the team noted their emergent ideas. Initial codes were identified systematically across the entire data set, and data relevant to each code were organized. Transcripts were then examined for possible themes, and a coding scheme was developed to reflect these themes. The investigative team systematically coded transcripts using the code book. Any disagreements encountered were resolved through discussion and by returning to the original text. NVivo software was used to assist in the management of textual data.

The verification of the findings was established with the following strategies: *credibility* attained through persistent observation, prolonged engagement in the field, and second interviews with young people; *transferability* via thick description of the context and each particular pathway; *dependability* through an audit trail established through observational and reflexive field notes and the tracking of decision making; and *confirmability* by way of team debriefing and analysis (Erlandson, Harris, Skipper, and Allen, 1993).

Results

Preliminary findings from this research revealed the dynamic complexity and inter-relatedness of the role of the family, school, community, treatment system and the illness experience in the pathway to mental health care (Boydell et al., 2008; Boydell, Addington, Gladstone, Stasiulus, and Volpe, 2000). Although each individual pathway was unique, common elements included: the difficulty of detecting psychosis on the part of GPs, psychiatrists, educators, peers, and family members; feelings of isolation and paranoia preventing youth from telling others about their experiences; the important role schools play in help seeking; and the pervasive lack of knowledge regarding psychosis. Research participants acknowledged that, if they had known that their symptoms might have been related to early signs of psychosis, they would have been more inclined to seek help earlier. The problem of stigma was also identified as a barrier to help seeking by both young people and their significant others. The importance of bringing knowledge about psychosis into the community, particularly into the school system, was a pervasive theme among all of the participants in the first episode study and was also identified in earlier research on rural mental health (Boydell, Stasiulis, Barwick, Greenberg, and Pong, 2008).

This chapter touches on some of the overall findings of this research but focuses primarily on the case study of a sixteen-year-old female with the pseudonym "Aalia." By closely examining a single case, we can see the context and specificity of how the identified themes play out. We chose to feature Aalia's case because it documented a less traumatic and, hence, what we would consider to be a more successful entry into the treatment system.[2] Unlike the other young people in the study, Aalia's route to care did not involve emergency hospital settings, the police, or incidents of self-harm. Her case highlights the ways in which various social processes and elements can interact in ways that both helped and impeded her pathway to care. It also reveals the integral role that schools play in directing young people to get appropriate help.

"Aalia"

Vignette

Aalia was sixteen at the time of interview and had been in the FEP program for six months. She lives at home with her parents and eighteen-year-old sister. She and her family emigrated from Pakistan when Aalia was in Grade 5.

Aalia's difficulties began in Grade 8. She was doing poorly academically, having trouble making friends, and feeling tired most of the time.

She cried for no reason and felt that people were making fun of her. Aalia's family thought that her behaviour might be related to culture shock.

Grade 9 was, in Aalia's words, an "excellent year." She did well and did not display any of the troubling behaviours from the previous year. However, beginning in Grade 10, behaviours of concern started to escalate. She became restless and agitated, isolating herself in her bedroom, watching television. Aalia told her teacher that people were bullying and making fun of her. Aalia was first referred to the guidance counsellor. Due to concerns that she was preoccupied with bullying and in need of psychological assistance, Aalia was then referred to the school social worker.

During this period, Aalia's family attributed her behaviour to laziness. This opinion was reinforced by the general practitioner's comments when he saw Aalia for a routine medical examination. He told her parents that she was lazy and "as long as school work is okay, why bother? Kids will be like that." At this time, Aalia did not tell the doctor she was hearing voices because she was afraid that he might harm her and her family.

Towards the end of Grade 10, Aalia abruptly informed the school social worker that she no longer needed therapy. Fearing that she might be planning to harm herself, the social worker notified the other school counsellors as well as her mother about her concerns. Communication among the counsellors and Aalia's mother increased considerably. The social worker credits Aalia's mother as being a "huge factor" in eventually getting her the proper help.

Beginning in April and continuing through May, Aalia's teacher brought her school-based journal entries about being bullied to the attention of the counsellors. Aalia herself told the teacher that many children were bullying her. In response to these messages and allegations, the school conducted a thorough investigation but could find no evidence of bullying. When Aalia's teacher reported other unusual behaviour to the counsellors, they began to suspect that there was something more going on.

A turning point for Aalia occurred when she learned about her poor exam results at the end of June. She became very upset and paranoid, fearing that her teacher was broadcasting her personal information to the government with the aim of sabotaging her future. As her mother says, "everything came out." This time when Aalia saw her general practitioner, she told him that she was hearing voices. The doctor immediately prescribed medication and made a referral for her to see a psychiatrist. In the meantime, Aalia's mother contacted the social worker about where to go for help now that they knew she was possibly experiencing psychiatric problems. The social worker gave Aalia's mother the contact information for the early psychosis intervention clinic from a brochure she had recently received at a presentation given by clinic staff. Shortly after her mother contacted the clinic, Aalia began attending the FEP program.

Recognizing Psychosis

Recognizing psychosis was pivotal to the help-seeking process in this case and across all cases. It poses the biggest challenge not only for those individuals closest to the young person but also for the young people themselves. Often psychotic symptoms are attributed to social, cultural, and personal factors. In Aalia's case, her behaviour was linked to culture shock (by her parents), laziness (by her parents and her GP), and being bullied (by her teachers). Consistent with the accounts of other study participants, Aalia recognized that something was not quite right, that "there was something wrong" with her. However, from looking at the topics she searched for on the Internet and the books she read, it does not seem that Aalia ever considered psychosis or a mental health disorder.

> *I knew there was something wrong with me...I was tired. I feel like people were making fun of me. (Aalia)*

> *I read books. I read "Life after Loss" and then I searched the Internet for "fear" and "frustration" and "self-centred." I thought that's what was wrong with me. (Aalia)*

Given the amount of time that young people spend in school, the potential for educators to detect psychosis is significant in the cases where young people are attending school. However, in most instances, the school plays a minimal role, if any role, in identifying a possible mental health issue. In contrast to the other cases in the study, the co-ordinated effort that Aalia's teachers and guidance counsellors made towards understanding her difficulties and getting her help led to her comparatively non-problematic entry into the early intervention clinic. However, Aalia's and her mother's belief that the school could have done more to help earlier points to the need for more education and awareness about psychosis.

> *She didn't think they could have found out real early because when I told my teacher that people were making fun of me, they aren't. She knows there is something wrong with me. She recommended me to see a counsellor. Maybe if they two had thought about what's happening, these two different stories, right? One is they are. One is they aren't. They could have found out at the beginning that I was suffering from psychosis. (Aalia)*

The teachers didn't notice anything. Even though she's withdrawing in the class and she's sitting near the window and she's behaving differently in the class. She's not participating. They don't care. If they're a good teacher they would have noticed. They don't care. (Mother)

They should notice this girl is not participating. Something is wrong. They should tell me so I can report to the doctor. (Mother)

I don't think we ever thought that she was having psychological problems. We just thought that she was just lonely. She was just disjoined from the group and distracted and we thought that, you know, just a student who needed to have some friends. Needed to feel a part of what was going on. It wasn't until she started to have different stories and things that we really started to be concerned. (Guidance counsellor)

Early analysis across the case studies reveals many failed attempts to get help within the health system itself. The inability of GPs, other health professionals, and even psychiatrists to recognize the signs and symptoms of mental illness have contributed to many missed opportunities for directing young people to appropriate services. Despite several visits, Aalia's GP was quick to dismiss her problems and did not probe further, attributing her behaviour to being lazy and typical of a teenager. It was not until Aalia disclosed that she was experiencing auditory hallucinations that her GP prescribed medication and immediately referred her to a psychiatrist.

We thought she was lazy like the doctor. We brought her to the doctor several times and the doctor said as long as she's doing school, why do you bother? (Mother)

We didn't get any help because when we told the doctor several times with some concerns, we would have expected some information from him. Even if he said, "Okay, you people are bothering me so much, I will send you to a psychiatrist." So, if she had visited the psychiatrist six months before, once we brought it to the notice of our family doctor, it would have been different maybe. (Mother)

The Very "Real" Nature of Symptoms

In looking back on their early experiences of psychosis, many participants stated that their symptoms seemed "real" and therefore contributed to the delay in help seeking. Since they believed their hallucinations and paranoia to be true, participants did not see them as being an indication of a mental health problem. Although they felt confused and frightened, they were reluctant to tell anyone about their experiences. Aalia's belief that her fellow students were "out to get her" affected what she told her guidance counsellor and, at one point, caused her to stop seeing her counsellor altogether. In addition, Aalia's paranoia around her GP, whom she felt wanted to harm her and was in a conspiracy with her mother, prevented her from telling the GP about the voices and thoughts she was experiencing.

> I feel like people think that I was thinking that because of the bullying I'm seeing her. If they know that I am seeing her, they will make more fun of me. So, I stopped. (Aalia)

> I was so sick when my mom told me to talk to a doctor. I even suspected the doctor might harm me... Sometimes I feel like my doctor is going to harm me, even my family doctor. (Aalia)

> So before the doctor used to ask, do you see anything? Do you hear voices? She used to say no. She never used to tell him because she was scared that if she told the doctor, the doctor may harm her. She had that kind of thinking. (Mother)

This element of realism also served to convince and distract others from recognizing that Aalia was experiencing symptoms of psychosis. For months, the school and Aalia's mother "completely believed" her claims about being bullied, because for Aalia it was real and, thus, her accounts were convincing. At the same time, it was only when Aalia's journal writings were discovered that the facade of realism crumbled, alerting her mother and teachers to the possibility that she was experiencing a mental health problem.

> An English teacher actually started to bring us some of the things that she wrote about. Her writings were sounding like they were autobiographical. So we found that she was talking about her own experiences but they were very strange experiences. Almost unrealistic, but she was sounding like they were real. (Guidance counsellor)

Awareness and Knowledge

The importance of being aware and knowledgeable about psychosis was reiterated across all cases. In Aalia's case, accounts by Aalia, her family, and her educators indicate that a lack of knowledge was responsible for the delay in acquiring appropriate help. Following a workshop presentation by the FEP clinic, the school social worker was able to assess Aalia's situation and direct her to appropriate care. The clinic information was passed on to Aalia's mother, leading to her entry into a FEP program.

Maybe if the teachers and counsellors are aware of it. Plus the students themselves. If they know there was a disease called psychosis. (Aalia)

But you know it took her (teacher) two years and she had nothing that she could really put her finger on and say, what's wrong with her? So you know, I think a little more education on early signs... we could have said she's not being bullied. She's making it up. (Guidance counsellor)

Certainly, just a little more knowledge would have helped all of us to be able to act a little earlier. (Guidance counsellor)

There's nothing to normalize it, to say this could happen. Maybe if they did presentations at the beginning... you know a part of health curriculum. Maybe if there was more emphasis, but they're also trying to teach other stuff... like emotional safety or mental health. But you know for the general population, it's still very much taboo. (Social worker)

Since the subject of mental health is very complex and the learning curve is so steep, it is also important to have ongoing education programs and to pay attention to detail when talking about mental health issues.

It'd be good for the information out there for ongoing education and I know that costs a lot of time and energy and resources but I think it's necessary because until you have to use or are faced with it, it's very hard to hold on to knowledge. (School social worker)

Besides a formal understanding of psychosis, having a personal relationship with the young person emerged as an integral factor in detecting psychosis and getting help. Since the school social worker was meeting with Aalia on a regular basis, she was able to get to know her better and build a relationship that eventually helped Aalia to reveal more about what was going on with her. When the network of support and communication expanded to include Aalia's mother, her teachers, and her guidance counsellor, they were able to, together, quickly detect the symptoms of psychosis and direct Aalia to appropriate help. Unlike other cases involving individuals over the age of sixteen, in which confidentiality issues prohibit communication between parents and medical professionals or school personnel, Aalia's mother was able to get more deeply involved in her case because her daughter was under the age of sixteen.

> *Her mother was a huge factor in making everything happen. (School social worker)*

Discussion

This chapter describes one case from a larger study that used a series of qualitative case studies to document the pathways to care for young people experiencing FEP. The focus on this case study allowed us to highlight the particularity of one "story" in order to provide individual contextual information about the pathway to mental health care. Aalia's pathway, in particular, underscores the importance of being able to recognize the symptoms of psychosis as a major influence in the help-seeking process. While Aalia acknowledged that there was a problem, like other young people in this study, she failed to understand it as a mental illness. Consequently, she and others in her network pursued explanations and solutions that diverted them from considering mental illness as a possibility. Aalia's case also highlights the ways in which the very real symptoms of psychosis interfere with help seeking, resulting in Aalia telling her story only "partially." Without full knowledge of the symptoms that young people are experiencing, it is very difficult for health professionals and educators to recognize that psychosis may be occurring. In this study, the individual's experience of psychotic symptoms as being "real" emerges as an important factor in the pathway to care, requiring further exploration.

A key facilitator in the help-seeking process in Aalia's case was the quality of the relationship with a significant other in the social network. Since the relationship was strong and characterized by trust, communication was enhanced and help was more readily accessed. This finding is supported by recent work by David and Ann Shier (2009) who highlight the critical role of family members and other close supporters and believe their potential contribution requires greater consideration. Rules around confidentiality that impede communication and relationship building among parents and school personnel also need to be rethought.

Aalia was actively looking for answers (via the Internet) to what was wrong from an early age (Grade 8), long before she spoke to her teacher about the bullying. Her mother believes that the teachers failed to recognize that something was wrong and to follow up on her withdrawal and behaviour changes. Mental health literacy is widely advocated in order to achieve better awareness of mental health issues, and it would ultimately lead to enhanced effectiveness of particular services and supports (Kelly,

Jorm, and Wright, 2007; McWilliams et al., 2010; Wright, McGorry, Harris, Jorm, and Pennell, 2006). Community educational interventions may promote help seeking by young people and their relatives (Brunet, Birchwood, Lester, and Thornhill, 2007). These interventions along with psycho-educational programs and mental health literacy campaigns must be rigorously studied in order to determine their impact. Further, the literature suggests that a lack of knowledge about mental illness perpetuates stigmatizing attitudes and behaviours, once again pointing to the importance of enhancing literacy and systemically determining the effectiveness of such initiatives (Pinfold, Toulmin, Thornicroft, Huxley, and Farmer, 2003; Rickwood, Deane, Wilson, and Chiarrochi, 2005). Current evidence suggests that educational programs could be developed with the aim of reducing the raised threshold for initiation of treatment, ultimately decreasing DUP (Franz et al., 2010).

Further analysis involving the multiple case study approach will allow us to focus on a holistic description and explanation and make use of an analytic comparison of cases, describing and explaining complex and interrelated group characteristics, patterns, structures, and processes. The NEM will allow continued exploration of the dynamic processes of service use and focus on young people and their interactions with others in their social network—all of whom may have a role in recognizing problems, influencing decisions, making referrals, and providing treatment and support.

Notes

1 At the time of writing data were available for eight of ten index cases and their significant others.
2 By less traumatic, we mean entry that was not characterized by crisis, namely, involvement with the police or via the emergency room.

References

Aday, L.A., and Andersen, R.M. (1974). *Behavioural model of families' use of health services* (Research Series no. 25). Chicago, IL: University of Chicago, Center for Health Administration Studies.

Addington, J. (2007). The promise of early intervention. *Early Intervention in Psychiatry, 1*(4), 294-307.

Addington, J., Leriger, E., and Addington, D. (2003). Symptom outcome one year after admission to an early psychosis program. *Canadian Journal of Psychiatry, 48*, 204-7.

Addington, J., van Mastrigt, S., and Addington, D. (2004). Duration of untreated psychosis: Impact on two-year outcome. *Psychological Medicine, 34*, 1-8.

Addington, J., van Mastrigt, S., Hutchinson, J., and Addington, D. (2002). Pathways to care: Help seeking behaviour in first episode psychosis. *Acta Psychiatrica Scand, 106,* 358-64.

Addington, J., Young, J., and Addington, D. (2003). Social outcome in early psychosis. *Psychological Medicine, 33,* 1119-24.

American Psychiatric Association. (2000). *Diagnostic and statistical manual of mental disorders DSM-IV* (4th edition). Washington, DC: American Psychiatric Association.

Andersen, R.M. (1995). Revisiting the behavioural model and access to medical care: Does it matter? *Journal of Health and Social Behaviour, 36,* 1-10.

Andersen, R.M., and Newman, J.R. (1973). Societal and individual determinants of medical care utilization in the United States. *Milbank Memorial Fund Quarterly, 51,* 95-124.

Birchwood, M. (1992). Early intervention in schizophrenia: Theoretical background and clinical strategies. *British Journal of Clinical Psychology, 31,* 257-78.

Birchwood, M., and Macmillan, F. (1993). Early intervention in schizophrenia. *Australian and New Zealand Journal of Psychiatry, 27,* 374-78.

Boydell, K.M., Addington, J., Gladstone, B., Goering, P., McCay, E., Krupa, T., Stasiulis, E., and Volpe, T. (2008). Using the network episode model as a framework to understand pathways to care for youth experiencing first episode psychosis. *Early Intervention in Psychiatry, 2*(1), A8.

Boydell, K.M., Addington, J., Gladstone, B., Stasiulis, E., and Volpe, T. (2000). Youth at ultra high risk for psychosis: A comprehensive examination of pathways to mental health care. *Early Intervention in Psychiatry, 2*(1), A7.

Boydell, K.M., Stasiulis, E., Barwick, M., Greenberg, N., and Pong, R. (2008). Challenges of knowledge translation in rural communities: The case of rural children's mental health. *Canadian Journal of Community Mental Health, 27*(1), 49-63.

Braun, V., and Clarke, V. (2006). Using thematic analysis in psychology. *Qualitative Research in Psychology, 3,* 77-101.

Brunet, K., Birchwood, M., Lester, H., and Thornhill, K. (2007). Delays in mental health service and duration of untreated psychosis. *Psychiatric Bulletin, 31,* 408-10.

Costello, E.J., Pescosolido, B.A., Angold, A., and Burns, B.J. (1998). A family network-based model of access to child mental health services. *Research in Community and Mental Health. 9,* 165-90.

Erlandson, D.A., Harris, E.L., Skipper, B., and Allen, S.D. (1993). *Doing naturalistic inquiry: A guide to methods.* Newbury Park, CA: Sage Publications.

Falloon, I.R.H. (1992). Early intervention for first episodes of schizophrenia: A preliminary exploration. *Psychiatry, 55:* 4-15.

Franz, L., Carter, T., Leiner, A.S., Bergner, E., Thompson, N.J., and Compton, M.T. (2010). Stigma and treatment delay in first-episode psychosis: A grounded theory study. *Early Intervention in Psychiatry, 4*(1), 47-56.

Ho, B., and Andreasen, N.C. (2001). Long delays in seeking treatment for schizophrenia (commentary). *The Lancet, 337,* 898-900.

Kelly, C.M., Jorm, A.F., and Wright, A. (2007). Improving mental health literacy as a strategy to facilitate early intervention for mental disorders (supplemental material). *Medical Journal of Australia, 187*(7), 26-30.

LeCompte, M.D., and Preissle, J. (1993). *Ethnography and qualitative design in educational research* (2nd edition). Orlando, FL: Academic Press.

Lieberman, J.A., and Fenton, W.S. (2000). Delayed detection of psychosis: Causes, consequences, and effect on public health. *American Journal of Psychiatry, 157*(11), 1727-30.

Lincoln, C., and McGorry, P. (1995). Who cares? Pathways to psychiatric care for young people experiencing a first episode of psychosis. *Psychiatric Services, 46*(11), 1166-71.

Lincoln, C., and McGorry, P. (1999). Pathways to care in early psychosis: Clinical and consumer perspectives. In P. McGorry and H.J. Jackson (Eds.), *The recognition and management of early psychosis: A preventive approach* (pp. 51-79). Cambridge: Cambridge University Press.

Lines, L. (2000). *An introduction to early psychosis intervention: Some relevant findings and emergent practices.* Toronto: Canadian Mental Health Association, National Office.

Malla, A., Norman, R., McLean, T., Scholten, D., and Townsend, L. (2003). A Canadian programme for early intervention in non-affective psychotic disorders. *Australian and New Zealand Journal of Psychiatry, 37*, 407-13.

McMaster University, Department of Psychiatry. (2003). *PsychDirect: Evidence-based mental health education and information.* Online: http://www.psychdirect.com/psychosis/.

McWilliams, S., Egan, P., Jackson, D., Renwick, L., Foley, S., Behan, C., and O'Callaghan, E. (2010). Caregiver psychoeducation for first-episode psychosis. *European Psychiatry, 25*(1), 33-38.

Morgan,C., Mallett, R., Hutchinson, G., and Leff, J. (2004). Negative pathways to psychiatric care and ethnicity: The bridge between social science and psychiatry. *Social Science and Medicine, 58*, 739-52.

Norman, R.M.G., and Malla, A. K. (2001) Duration of untreated psychosis: A critical examination of the concept and its importance. *Psychological Medicine, 31*, 381-400.

Patton, M. (1990). *Qualitative evaluation and research methods.* Newbury Park, CA: Sage Publications.

Pescosolido, B.A. (1992). Beyond rational choice: The social dynamics of how people seek help. *American Journal of Sociology, 97*, 1096-1138.

Pescosolido, B.A. (1998). Social networks and patterns of use among the poor with mental health problems in Puerto Rico. *Medical Care, 36*(7), 1057-72.

Pinfold, V., Toulmin, H., Thornicroft, G., Huxley, P., and Farmer, P. (2003). Reducing psychiatric stigma and discrimination: Evaluation of educational interventions in UK secondary schools. *British Journal of Psychiatry, 182*, 342-46.

Richardson, L. (2001). Seeking and obtaining mental health services: What do parents expect? *Archives of Psychiatric Nursing, 15*(5), 223-31.

Rickwood, D., Deane, F.P., Wilson, C.J., and Ciarrochi, J. (2005). Young people's help-seeking for mental health problems (supplemental material). *Australian e-Journal for the Advancement of Mental Health*, 4(3), 1-34.

Shiers, D., Rosen, A., and Shiers, A. (2009). Beyond early intervention: Can we adopt alternative narratives like "Woodshedding" as pathways to recovery in schizophrenia? *Early Intervention in Psychiatry*, 3(3), 163-71.

Spitzer, R.L., Williams, J.B.W., Gibbons, M., and First, M.B. (1992). The structured clinical interview for DSM –III-R (SCID). *Archives of General Psychiatry*, 49(8), 624-29.

Wright, A., McGorry, P.D., Harris, M.G., Jorm, A.F., and Pennell, K. (2006). Development and evaluation of a youth mental health community awareness campaign: The Compass Strategy. *BMC Public Health*, 6, 215.

Yin, R.K. (1994). *Case study research: Design and methods* (Applied Social Research Methods Series Volume 5). Newbury Park, CA: Sage Publications.

2

Help-Seeking Experiences of Youth with First Episode Psychosis: A Research-Based Dance Production

Katherine M. Boydell, Siona Jackson, and John S. Strauss

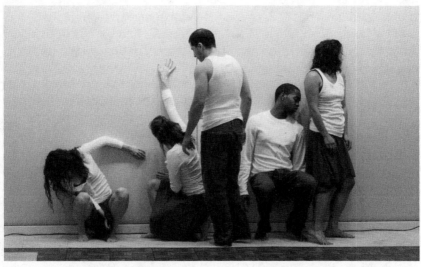

The Anguish of Psychosis. Performance of Dancing the Data, for the symposium "Hearing Voices: The Utilization of Qualitative Research in First Episode Psychosis," October 2007. Photograph by Ashley Hutcheson. Image reprinted with permission of the photographer.

Background/Literature Review

Arts-informed research has begun to capture the attention of a number of researchers. Interest in arts-based research methods has grown over recent years, as one consequence of a comprehensive epistemology that recognizes different forms of knowledge (Reason, 1988, 1994). Of particular interest is the demonstrated potential of visual methodologies in the study of health and illness, particularly the ways in which participants interpret, give meaning to, and make sense of their experiences (Harrison, 2002). Visual methodologies are a powerful tool for eliciting individual experiences and thus offer researchers new dimensions from which to view a phenomenon (Harper, 1998; Rapport, 2004). Arts-related methods problematize the relationship between knowledge and power in our society, exposing knowledge as socially constructed and creating open texts that strive to give voice to those people often silenced. When speaking about particular issues and experiences, words are often sadly insufficient to convey the passion and emotion felt: "Voices seem muted and inauthentic" (Rogers and Babinski in Sparkes, 2003, p. 417). Arts-informed research makes scholarly work accessible to broader and more diverse communities through the use of various art forms.

Few qualitative studies move beyond passive dissemination—for example, peer reviewed manuscripts (Bochner and Ellis, 2003; Keen and Todres, 2006). Traditional methods of dissemination frequently confine audiences to fellow academics (Barnes, Clouder, Pritchard, Highes, and Purkis, 2003) and pose an obstacle to research use, often separating researchers from practice and action (Mullen, 2003; Sandelowski, Trimble, Woodard, and Barroso, 2006). Universities and granting bodies are becoming increasingly responsive to demands that research activities be more relevant or community-centred and more accessible to the wider social community (Boydell, 2004; Cole, 2002). The literature in the field of health and education abounds with studies that focus on getting research out to a broader audience. Qualitative researchers have increasingly turned to alternative modes of research dissemination that are commonly associated with the humanities and arts, in part to address this problem (Ellis and Bochner, 1996; Finley, 2005; Knowles and Cole, 2008; Madison and Hamera, 2006; Norris, 1997). The turn to more artistic forms has also formed in response to the "crisis of representation" in qualitative research and the inadequacies of the traditional scientific research report to represent the lives of research participants (Smith, 2004, p. 962-63).

Photography, music, dance, poetry, video installations, dramatic monologues, and theatrical performances have recently been added to the strategies that qualitative researchers employ (Bagley and Cancienne, 2001, 2002; Bochner and Ellis, 2003; Cancienne, 2008). Those individuals engaging in this new "performative social science" are often altering these boundaries or moving beyond them. These qualitative investigators are intrepidly developing arts-based research methods and dissemination techniques with the goal of reaching more diverse and wider audiences.

Arts-informed methodologies bring together the "systematic and rigorous qualities of scientific inquiry with the artistic and imaginative qualities of the arts" (Cole and Knowles, 2001; Knowles and Cole, 2008). Arts-informed research has the potential to reach out beyond academia to the communities beyond (Cole and Knowles, 2001). In fact, there is an increasing scholarly literature on the use of art as a foundation for inquiry, as a means for producing knowledge and contributing to human understanding, and as a way of representing the complexities of the human experience (Gray, 2003, 2004; Knowles and Cole, 2008; Mason, 2005; Rapport, Wainwright, and Elwyn, 2005). Many research products now disregard the usual boundaries and forms of social scientific writing and include autoethnographies, poetry, performance texts, layered accounts, and visual representations (Bochner and Ellis, 2003; Denzin, 1997; Ellis and Bochner, 1996; Keen and Todres, 2006; Nisker, Martin, Bluhm, and Daar, 2006; Plummer, 2001; Richardson, 1992). In addition, the arts-informed educational community has also contributed much to the field (Barone, 2000; Cole, 2002; Eisner, 1991, 1993, 1997; Perselli, 2005) by demonstrating the power of alternative media in communicating research messages.

Similar work has recently proliferated in the medical community, exploring a wide variety of health care issues. Steven Keen and Les Todres (2006, 2007) reviewed sixty-two texts using non-traditional dissemination strategies in qualitative health research. These studies included modes of dissemination closely associated with media and art genres—that is, research-based theatre/ethno-drama (Gray, 2000, 2003; Gray, Fitch, Phillips, Labrecque, and Fergus, 2000; Gray and Sinding, 2002; Gray et al., 2000; Mienczakowski, 1995, 1996, 1997, 2003; Morgan, Rolfe, and Mienczakowski, 1993; Rolfe, Mienczakowsli, and Morgan, 1995), three-dimensional multimedia presentations (Cole and McIntyre, 2003, 2004, 2006), dance (Bagley and Cancienne, 2001), patchwork quilts including audio and photographs (Brackenbury, 2004), documentary film (Tilleczek et al., 2004), and poetic texts (Glesne, 1997; O'Connor, 2001; Richardson, 1992). Their review identified that the studies moved beyond the most traditional of passive techniques (the journal article) to disseminate their findings. For example, a smaller subset of authors relied on an empirical foundation for dissemination, and three projects attempted to address the communicative concern of qualitative research findings by evaluating their impact (Gray, Fitch, Phillips, Labrecque, and Fergus, 2000; Gray, Fitch, Labrecque, and Greenburg, 2003; Mienczakowski, 1995, 2003). These three examples move beyond dissemination that traditionally serves academic communities and provide scholarly examples of the dissemination and impact of qualitative research findings on practice, policy, and people. The purpose is not to weaken or replace the scholarship of either qualitative research or the peer-reviewed journal manuscript (Morse, 2004). Rather, in communicating findings from qualitative data, researchers have a wide range of (re)presentational approaches and formats to select from that best fit their research purposes (Sandelowski, 1998). This array of approaches offers the potential to broaden the perspective of what counts as knowledge and induces different ways of knowing and understanding (Simons and McCormack, 2007). The *Handbook of the Arts in Qualitative Research* by Gary Knowles and Ardra Cole (2008) offers a comprehensive discussion of the arts in research across numerous disciplines in the social sciences as well as a range of examples. One of the areas of arts-informed inquiry that remains relatively under-represented is dance (Bagley and Cancienne, 2001).

The purpose of this chapter is to describe the partnership between a scientist (Katherine Boydell, researcher) and artist (Siona Jackson, choreographer) who co-created an eleven-minute dance performance based on the study entitled *Youth Experiencing First Episode Psychosis: A Comprehensive Evaluation of Pathways to Care*, which was funded by the Canadian Institutes of Health Research (Boydell, Addington, Gladstone, Stasiulis, and Volpe 2008; Boydell et al., 2008). The goal was to explicitly draw on the evocative power of the arts in enhancing representation, generating new insights, and increasing understanding of youth experiences of help seeking (Daykin, 2004). The chapter ends with a commentary by psychiatrist John S. Strauss.

Telling Our Stories

Katherine Boydell, Scientist

I wanted to move away from a strictly text-based interpretation of the data and give privilege to an embodied representation of the data. For many years, I have been interested in the ways in which we communicate our research findings to a wide variety of stakeholders—specifically, the use of creative arts in the design, process, analysis, interpretation, and communication of research results. How can the creative arts draw out and depict the essential findings of research and promote useable knowledge and understanding? What are the connections that exist between art and science? Although on the surface, these two disciplines seem extremely different and have traditionally been conceptualized as separate realms, they both embrace and celebrate the importance of innovation and creativity. As Paul Wainwright and Frances Rapport (2007) have noted, the artistic creative process and qualitative research are inextricably bound up with recurrent themes of form, structure, content, and meaning. Artist and researcher take experience and seek to translate it into a form that others can experience and interpret.

For many years now, I have been pondering the use of the arts to aid in communicating research with young people experiencing psychosis. Dance, for me, was of particular interest—a blending of my two worlds—that of scientist with my immersion in the dance world (via three "dancing" daughters). I found myself continuously moved by the power of dance to communicate a story—for me, dance was a metaphor for the qualitative research process—its parallels with the aims of qualitative research were many. Was it possible to develop visual ways to communicate research findings about multi-faceted subjects such as psychosis? How does one move from a written language to body language? Could it challenge us to engage differently with the data and to see differently? To take a subject matter and a form (psychosis and dance) and combine them has the potential to extend the intensity and depth of meaning.

I met Siona several years ago, as she was a guest choreographer at my daughter's dance studio. I was moved by the way she worked with the dancers, by her creativity, and by her ability to engage both the dancers and the audience with her innovative choreography. Needless to say, it was her dance creations that consistently won awards. Over coffee, I discussed with Siona the idea of co-creating a dance performance that would be based on the results emerging from my research team's work in first episode psychosis (FEP). I shared my belief that the choreographic process and the research process were similar in terms of the central role of interpretation. She acknowledged that using dance as a communication tool for representing data on early psychosis would create an opportunity for people to think about research on psychosis in an accessible, creative, and thoughtful way.

We talked at length about the ability of dance to explore knowledge physically, emotionally, and mentally, allowing the audience to experience the material immediately without analyzing it. When Siona stated that dance has the capacity to capture individual stories, revisit an experience, and create a voice that we do not have words for but somehow understand in a gesture, a glance, or silent moment, I knew that we could make something happen. Several years following this chat in the coffee shop, an opportunity presented itself in terms of a venue and resources to allow for the creation of the dance. I was the organizer of an international symposium on qualitative inquiry in FEP and had some "knowledge translation" funds in a research slush account, which allowed me to engage with Siona, the dancers, and the musician. The dancer can capture an embodied understanding—glimpses of the indescribable and unknowable elements of lived experience. I believed that "dancing the data" had the potential to evoke different ways of knowing and understanding. Artistic expression is one way of capturing the particularity and the universality of a person's experience—something we are always doing as qualitative researchers.

Siona Jackson, Choreographer

My world is dance—ever since I was three. I took classes upon classes of different types for years: "1 and a 2, 3 and a 4...stretch your arms, point your feet, 5, 6, 7, 8! Smile!" I was constantly developing a skill that connected my thoughts and feelings into movement. This movement allowed me to communicate to the audience, and soon I found out that being a dancer is what I loved to do. A defining moment for me in my life was when I forgot my solo choreography on stage—yes, stage fright! I ended up running off stage into my teacher's arms and crying purely because my mind would not let me remember my work. My parents later told me that when that happens just make it up—the audience will not know the difference—but, whatever you do, stay on stage and finish! And, sure enough, during my next solo, my fears came back, and in the middle of the movement with 300 people staring at me my mind went blank for a split second. But then I did it, I starting making it up—I bridged a gap and felt fearless and danced that solo with more energy than I ever had! That day taught me that there is power in moving an audience and to trust myself on stage.

As my career developed in dance, I explored choreography and found great satisfaction in telling stories through movement no matter what the subject. This is what choreographers are to me—storytellers. Creating live pictures that evoke an experience. Music plays a large role in this experience and often completes the choreography like a frame around a picture. Music can be shaped and mixed like choreography and can evoke the same emotion without movement or words. This is why it is such a powerful mix. As a choreographer, I seek projects that involve a certain amount of importance and intelligence and that can reflect what our (my) environment is saying and or experiencing. Dance choreography has a unique way of expressing information and emotion that allows the spectator to have a personal connection to the material. Simple gestures can say so much.

I was inspired by Katherine. She had this gut instinct that "dance creation" is a very valuable vehicle for translating research. This notion stemmed from her experience watching and supporting her children dance, perform, and develop their creative ability. In my observation, Katherine understands the "connection" of the two worlds and understands that there is a bridge that connects them and can help to identify deeper findings and understanding.

Conceptualizing the Project

Katherine Boydell, Scientist
My goal was to take some of the thematic findings from my team's study on *Youth Experiencing First Episode Psychosis: A Comprehensive Examination of Pathways to Care* and illuminate these findings through a physical embodied representation as well as the use of textual devices to aid in interpretation. My regular meetings with Siona were treated in typical "research" style over the development phase, as I audiotaped all of our meetings in order to document the process of developing the dance. When Siona asked me to share some of the themes that emerged—actual words or a series of words—to help convey the research findings to her and to inspire the choreography, I felt confident and trusted that she would represent the results that were emerging in a meaningful and evocative manner. I provided Siona with words that represented a dialectic of sorts but that occurred along a continuum in the stories of the experiences of young people and their significant others in our study as they navigated and negotiated pathways to care (see Figure 1).

During the development of the choreography and at rehearsals, my research team (Brenda Gladstone, Elaine Stasiulis, and Tiziana Volpe) and I were able to communicate some of the main messages emerging from our study of FEP to Siona, the dancers, and the musician who was responsible for creating the musical score in an iterative manner. Following an overview of the definition of psychosis and the general field of early intervention in psychosis, we highlighted the richness of the in-depth case studies that involved qualitative interviews with ten different young people and everyone they had identified in their network who played a role in their

FIGURE 1

normal—abnormal
accepting—resisting/rejecting
reaching out—withdrawing/holding back
losing control—gaining control
active—passive
hope—despair
coping—collapse
darkness—light
heavy—light
denial—claiming of
crisis—transformation
weak—strong
layered stories/fractured stories
changed identity/new identity
interruption/disruption/interference

pathway to care, whether it was a facilitative role or not. We talked about the complexity of the pathway and the fact that although every young person's pathway was unique there were common experiences across all of the cases. There was a great deal of help-seeking activity, and this process involved subtle and not so subtle changes (Boydell et al., 2006a, 2006b; Boydell, Gladstone, and Volpe, 2006). There were a number of persons and multiple systems involved in these help-seeking activities, but they rarely communicated with each other. There were many failed attempts at accessing appropriate services and supports, and these efforts were conceptualized as "missed opportunities" (Gladstone, Volpe, and Boydell, 2007).

I received confirmation from the research manager of the Ethics Board at the Hospital for Sick Children to share some of the "anonymized" transcripts with Siona who was regarded as a new member of the team. Her reading of the raw data and subsequent discussions with our research team helped her to further immerse herself in the study and gain a greater understand of the lived experience of seeking help from the perspective of young people. I felt the tension of trying to balance my input in the product with a need to provide space for Siona to use her creativity—I knew that I had to "let go" and give her the freedom to work with the data we had shared with her.

Siona Jackson, Choreographer

This project was just the right venue into which to inject dance. Unknown territory excites choreographers as it gives them a lot of room to explore and develop a new way of interpreting movement. Allowing physical movement to be the voice for such a weighty subject had my mind spinning as Katherine described her vision. Katherine had expressed her vision of using dance as a communication tool to create impact and to bring an emotional and human experience to the audience of her fellow peers and students.

I constantly reminded myself that the purpose of the dance was to communicate what could not be described or felt with the text or research journals—possibly knowledge that was untold or not sensed. The excitement of the impact, curiosity, and an alternative way of delivering research exposes new findings or pathways to findings. I understood Katherine's desire that this piece not be "over-performed" but, rather, "felt" in a way that needed to be human and honestly experienced. It was important to me not to turn this dance into an entertainment performance on the program but, rather, to express and communicate as closely as we could the experience of these young people seeking help as described in their transcribed narratives. This goal required less "technical movement" and more "character movement." There was a need to focus on the emotional journey and to have the movement reflect this process.

I felt that Katherine trusted me right from the very beginning with all that was involved in building this piece. She left me the room to interpret my own vision alongside hers. This trust made me nervous and excited at the same time. It made me feel nervous as I struggled to understand Katherine's world of writing journals, conducting research, and constantly discussing these ideas with her colleagues and research team—using terminology that sometimes went over my head! I kept reminding myself that I was someone who had analyzed, observed, and produced in physical form, using the body and music, a world that was used to being expressed in text. It was fascinating and I have to admit I was amazed at how much Katherine had read and recorded. Her computer desktop was packed with files with no room to spare! The more Katherine and I chatted and the more I read and found out, the more it made perfect sense that our worlds could come together and fuse well. Research and dance are processes that are very similar to one another. They share the actions of analyzing, reviewing, breaking down, developing, testing, suggesting, and creating.

The six-month timeline was very generous and healthy to accomplish what needed to be done. I wondered how I was to begin. Question everything! Listen, talk, try a move; listen, talk, try a move; brainstorm, envision, move; brainstorm, envision, move. I wondered what was going to be the best way to accomplish this endeavour? How was I going to develop the material to the point of dancing? I planned to use the transcripts of the tape-recorded interviews of the case studies that had been conducted. I would take the data from these case studies and individually examine them to create a story in six parts. I began this process by breaking down three specific interviews. I was reading and listening for emotional cues—shifts in the nature of the words—and I was hearing the responses of the people conducting the interviews, all coming from the page. This work started the wheels turning, and I brought in my dance assistant (Courtnae Bowman) and a composer (Tim Isherwood). Then Katherine and her research team came in to one of those early rehearsals where I witnessed a noteworthy relationship that developed between the creative and research teams. The research team's involvement was crucial in that it provided feedback into the way in which the performance was evolving and shaping the ultimate product. The meetings held between the dancers, musician, choreographer, and research team offered a lens into both worlds—the dancers were able to ask their questions about the subject matter and the research team could see the ways in which a thematic concept from the study was integrated into the dance movements. This feedback inspired me to condense my original idea of including six parts to focusing on only the three case studies that represented the key concepts and themes inherent in all of them. It was at this point that the project took off.

The Product

About the Script

I decided to use a script to keep track of all of the activity presented in the performance to provide a reference of what we were trying to get across—an organizational tool to communicate clearly. The reason that the script was required was a result of the multiple meetings, interviews, articles, and workshops that occurred, which were, at times, somewhat overwhelming. It helped to condense this information into a story-like dance that would educate an audience and not overwhelm them. The process unfolded from identifying the symptoms (a key activity since the symptoms represent reaction, emotion, and care—which we can dance) to relating to the people in the interviews, building character backgrounds, and, finally, condensing the entire research project into a "general focus" that would provide the highest impact. The script marked out where the props would go (the bench), where the dancers would be, what type of mood was being expressed, what the musical and dancer cues were, what emotions were to be portrayed, such as breathing. Once the basic script was in place, I had the freedom to layer the stories and the choreography.

Although the choreography was not recorded on the script, the blocking (patterns of the dancers) was. I relied on the dancers to memorize the movement, which was recorded from time to time on video. The script also

FIGURE 2: SAMPLE SEGMENT

SCRIPT: HEARING VOICES

OPENING:
Prop needed: Marker
Spacing:
Coutnae: centre stage, facing downstage left
Shavar: downstage right of Courtnae, facing downstage left
Nicola: downstage left of Courtnae and right of Nicola, facing downstage right
Lisa: upstage right of Courtnae, facing Jeff
Mariano: offstage, coming on to start movement—stars onstage right beside Courtnae
Mariano: writes the word 'freak' on Courtnae. He passes the marker to Courtnae. He then molds to others.
Courtnae: watches the writing and then looks up. Whispers on Mariano's writing movement.
Others: Whisper their voices when he is writing and then turn and look away from Courtnae when she looks up.

served as a communication tool for the composer—in our sessions, we built the score from the beginning, so that the ideas on the page inspired the music. Once the script was complete, it helped us when we met with the research team, as we knew exactly where to tweak or edit the content and when to add more movement to the dance (see Figure 2).

The Cast

Developing the cast was a simple process. I knew who I wanted for a while and added a couple more dancers by the end. All of the dancers were chosen based on their individual presence on the stage and by the way in which they were able to deliver the choreography. We did have feedback to say that the dancers represented the case study well by their diversity in terms of gender, colour, culture, and personalities. The culture factor was not a conscious choice at the time of hiring.

The Costumes

The costumes were very simple and reflective of the message, the environment, and the setting. The use of a black marker to write on the white t-shirts became a highlight of the opening act as the dancers scribbled key words from the study themes onto one another.

The Music

Initially, recorded music was considered for the dance, however, eventually it was felt that the experience was not asking for this sort of music. We decided that it needed to be original and that is why the musician Tim Isherwood was brought in to compose the original score. Our creation process was a long one, and it took more than 200 hours of studio time to produce the eleven-minute piece. The music was inspired by the transcript data, discussions with the research team and the dancers, and video footage from the rehearsals. An iterative process ensued, one of going back and forth to tweak, edit, redo, and experiment with sounds that reflected the choreography.

The Audience

The audience played a key role in the creation of the dance. The main audience for the performance consisted of academics—psychiatrists, physicians, research scientists and their students, and other health care practitioners working with youth who were experiencing FEP. The audience was international in scope and included participants from across Canada, the United States, the United Kingdom, and Australia.

Exploring the Impact of Research-Based Dance

In exploring the potential of alternate forms of representation for illuminating the worlds we wish to understand, it is important to measure the audience response. In a trans-disciplinary world, we are working outside conventional boundaries and uncovering moments that may be difficult to define or categorize by engaging with new experiences and improvising unorthodox combinations of knowledge. It was critical for us to garner the immediate audience response to the performance. The dance was performed to two very unique audiences: choreographers, dancers, musicians, and actors from the arts world in a rehearsal held the day prior to the symposium and the health care practitioners and researchers present at the symposium. In both instances, spectators were asked to take a few minutes to write their reaction to the dance on a "sticky note" provided to them. They were told that it could be a word, a series of words, or a sentence or two. In the case of the symposium, there were several large poster boards outside of the room and the audience members affixed their responses to the boards on their way out to the break. In this way, the audience was able to see how others responded and this encouraged further dialogue throughout the day. There were also additional opportunities for the audience to provide their feedback—at the end of the day via an evaluation form and following the symposium via e-mail. Some of the questions the audience was asked to consider included: Is artistic expression an effective means of capturing the particularity and universality of a person's experience? Does this performance have the potential to serve as a catalyst for dialogue and collaboration? Did it contribute to an empathic participation in the lives of others? Is this an effective knowledge translation strategy?

Sixty individuals responded on their sticky notes after witnessing the performance. Responses were overwhelmingly positive and addressed the importance of pursuing this genre to communicate research results to a wide variety of audiences. Some of these responses included:

This was such a great public display of subjective experiences through an art medium. I believe this to be a powerful method to educate and sensitize about psychosis, but especially to fight against stigma!

Pain-trying-Cycles-Alone/Not-(dis)connect-Break/broken/flee
So much pain that as a professional I CAN'T fell w/ every person b/c I'll drown but this reminds me why I do my job. Reminds me HOW I should—That words aren't enough to understand.

Extremely interesting way of conveying the findings of the study. Provides a human face to this illness and the use of words, music, sound and dance is powerful. Evokes emotional response to subject matter.

> *touching,*
> > *mind to heart,*
> *connection,*
> > *inspiration,*
> > > *transformation,*
> > > > *transcendence.*

Further research is thus required in order to explore the reception, meaning making, and impact that results for audience members who witness dance as a form of research dissemination. Such efforts would help to refine and deepen the research that uses this genre. Dance-based inquiry has limitations since the themes that are used in the choreographic process be may deemed to be selective and subjective. The shaping of the performance clearly relied on artistic and aesthetic appeal and utilized a particular lens or perspective. In spite of these drawbacks, though, transforming research data into an artistic performance allows opportunities for the emotional to be observed through body, gesture, music, and voice. Such a goal is not directly accessible in other forms of research.

Reflections

Katherine Boydell, Scientist

This collaboration between artists and scientists has been a meaningful and exciting one on so many different levels. I hope it will act as a catalyst for interdisciplinary and trans-disciplinary collaboration. I think that there is great potential to use educational and interactional formats that could be designed as companion programming to build understanding and awareness of early psychosis in young people and to share these empirical research findings with a wide variety of stakeholder audiences. There is widely documented need for mental health literacy in a wide variety of settings, particularly in schools. Despite efforts to increase awareness about FEP and mental illness in general, strategies to educate young people, their families, and the wider community have been largely unsuccessful. The stigma and discrimination associated with mental illness prevents young people from seeking help and generates derogatory, stereotyped reactions from society as a whole (Thornicroft, 2006). This problem calls for creative, innovative, and provocative strategies. Arts-informed research provides a platform from which to begin a dialogue with different and diverse audiences and has the potential of moving them towards new ways of understanding and knowing (O'Connor, 2001). The use of the arts, including lectures, panels, interactive workshops, "talkback" sessions, hands-on experience, town hall meetings, and publications, may be one way. I hope to attain funding to pursue further development and research exploring the impact of arts-informed inquiry. It is important to consider adding the involvement and voice of young people and their families to these endeavours. Dance offers a different way into the experiences of health, illness, and healthcare and the ways in which the participants themselves interpret, give meaning to, and make sense of their experiences. This arts-informed methodology will contribute to our understanding of the pathways to mental health care.

Siona Jackson, Choreographer

What stood out the most, and was most important for me as a choreographer, was sharing the steps of the process with several people (Katherine and her research team). The creative process is regarded as a sacred space and one that tends to be private, but I loved feeling exposed, having the work viewed, and receiving feedback as the process unfolded. What a joy it was to bring data and research results into a live experience! It was amazing that you could watch something that honours the research, respects the individuals that took part in the study, and creates an impact with art. The excitement of impact, curiosity, and an alternative way of delivering research exposes new findings or paths to these findings.

Our movements speak—often louder than our words. Our bodies hold our lives' experiences and memories, and a gesture or posture can betray grief, happiness, tension, pain, joy, desire, enthusiasm, or fear—despite our verbal denials. Bridging these two worlds created a ripple effect for both of us. I can see dance as a valuable tool in research for many different outlets. I am presently creating a performance for cancer—that focuses on living life and using the shock of having cancer as a tool to promote yourself and your body's health to live beyond it. I feel a little more connected to understanding psychosis, something that I did not reflect much on before this project. Knowledge is power, and it was felt by all of my dancers as well as myself. The entire process resulted in great satisfaction. I know I will continue to create work that involves this type of process.

John Strauss, Scientist

I have spent my life doing "real science" in the mental health field, but I just wish you could have seen this dance program. I think it would have moved you greatly but also provided a much broader view than is usually accepted regarding the range of inputs we need in order to have a truly *human science* in the mental health field. Although my early psychiatric training was psychodynamic, including a great deal of intensive work with schizophrenic patients, and although I valued that work, I also longed during those early years for something more like real science. So I was delighted when I joined the World Health Organization's International Pilot Study of Schizophrenia where we really attended to the reliability of our data, its validity, issues of sampling, operational definitions, and careful statistical analysis. Throughout my research on the course of illness and diagnosis, I have always been in the enviable position of doing both a sizable number of the research interviews as well as the data analysis and theory. Over the years, it has become increasingly possible not only to test various psychiatric hypotheses such as the then accepted hypothesis that people with schizophrenia never improve (we showed in the early 1970s that they often do) but also to notice that there has been a vast amount of data about patients' subjective experience that was systematically excluded from our field primarily because it was too difficult to measure and to define operationally. Believing increasingly that it was bad science to ignore a huge mass of data that was so obviously important, or to deceive ourselves by the belief that "we do it already" when listening to patients' accounts since we clearly were not, I came to feel that it is absolutely essential, as Pierre Main de Biran noted in 1814, that if we are to study humans we must find better approaches to deal with their (and our) subjectivity. Increasingly, it has appeared to me that Ludwig Feuerbach was correct when he (and, subsequently, many others) held that there were two kinds of knowledge. These have been called by many names such as subjective and objective, or experiential and discursive, or knowing and understanding, but the basic idea seems valid, that especially in a science dealing with humans we require both kinds of knowledge and neither can be substituted for the other. In understanding mental health and illness, for example, the experiences of anguish, hope, courage, determination, fear, and even being cared about and/or taken seriously by another person can simply not be adequately captured under a concept such as "quality of life." And these important and sometimes subtle subjective experiences appear to have a major impact on the course of disorder and perhaps even on its etiology. We have proposed therefore that our field needs to pay more attention to information that is available through the arts so that we can do justice to human subjectivity in accompaniment with the sophisticated methods that have been developed for dealing objectively with human phenomena. I have published, often in French journals where there is more interest in this possibility, various articles and studies about how careful consideration of the arts teaches important things about mental illness and health.

Nevertheless, when Katherine mentioned that our conference would begin with a dance performance, I was skeptical. The traditional scientist within me figured that such a thing might be cute, or even beautiful, but it would probably also be irrelevant to our mission. However, Siona and her dance group then performed, and the dancing and music were enthralling and very powerful. How to tell you how and why? I can best do it, but so incompletely, by trying to describe my experience of the performance. Previously during my life, through carrying out extensive and intensive treatment including psychological, social, and medication approaches as well as through research interviews—often repeated interviews carried out with the same patients over a period of four years or longer—I have known literally hundreds of adults and adolescents with the entire range of psychotic diagnoses. I have tried to listen to them to get a sense of what their experiences involved, and I believed that I had arrived at a rather good understanding of those experiences. Yet there was something about that dance performance that washed away my previous assurance of the adequacy of my knowledge as well as my initial skepticism. This performance allowed me to feel "oh that is what psychosis can be like." For example, one of the problems with symptom-rating forms and, surprisingly, even with dramatic productions is their huge tendency to oversimplify, to put the aspects of being psychotic in a little box and indicate that this is what it is. Even the great Betty Davis in the movie Juarez, playing the wife of the betrayed Maximilian, as she becomes psychotically paranoid, does not get it. There is in psychosis a mixture of normal and "psychotic," of disorganized and organized, of effective and incompetent, that I am sure is essential to our understanding of psychotic processes and yet is systematically missed by our theories, our concepts, and our treatments. One of the many things that the dancers and their music conveyed was a feeling of these subtle mixtures. I am not sure how they did that, but they got it and they communicated it to us. It is now up to the advance of our human science to figure out how they did it and what else in the realm of patient subjectivity they captured and then to elaborate on how that can help us better understand our patients and develop more adequate theories and treatments.

References

Bagley, C., and Cancienne, M.B. (2001). Educational research and inter-textual forms of (re)presentation: The case for dancing the data. *Qualitative Inquiry*, 7(2), 221-37.

Bagley, C., and Cancienne, M.B. (2002). Educational research and inter-textual forms of (re)presentation: The case for dancing the data. In C. Bagley and M.B. Cancienne (Eds.), *Dancing the data* (pp. 3-19). New York: Peter Lang.

Barnes, V., Clouder, D.L., Pritchard, J., Highes, C., and Purkis, J. (2003). Deconstructing dissemination: Dissemination as qualitative research. *Qualitative Research*, 3(2), 147-64.

Barone, T. (2000). *Aesthetics, politics, educational inquiries: Essays and examples.* New York: Peter Lang.

Bochner, A.P., and Ellis, C. (2003). An introduction to the arts and narrative research: Art as inquiry. *Qualitative Inquiry*, 9(4), 506-14.

Boydell, K.M. (2004). *What counts? Toward a new definition of scholarship.* Toronto: Hospital for Sick Children, Population Health Sciences.

Boydell, K.M., Addington, J., Gladstone, B., Goering, P., McCay, E., Krupa, T., Stasiulis, E., and Volpe, T. (2006a). Youth experiencing first episode psychosis: A comprehensive examination of pathways to mental health care (supplemental material). *Schizophrenia Research*, 86, 116.

Boydell, K.M., Addington, J., Gladstone, B., Goering, P., McCay, E., Krupa, T., and Volpe, T. (2006b). Understanding help-seeking delay in first psychosis prodrome: A secondary analysis of the perspectives of young people (supplemental material). *Schizophrenia Research*, 86, 124.

Boydell, K.M., Addington, J., Gladstone, B., Goering, P., McCay, E., Krupa, T., Stasiulis, E., and Volpe, T. (2008). Using the network episode model as a framework to understand pathways to care for youth experiencing first episode psychosis (supplemental material). *Early Intervention in Psychiatry*, 2(1), A8.

Boydell, K.M., Addington, J., Gladstone, B., Stasiulis, E., and Volpe, T. (2008). Youth at ultra high risk for psychosis: A comprehensive examination of pathways to mental health care (supplemental material). *Early Intervention in Psychiatry,* 2(1), A7.

Boydell, K.M., Gladstone, B., and Volpe, T. (2006). Understanding help seeking delay in the prodrome: Perspectives of young people. *Psychiatric Rehabilitation Journal*, 30(1), 54-60.

Brackenbury, J. (2004). Pulling together the threads: Boundaries, silences and the continuum of care among women in families. *Arts-informed*, 4(1), 19-20. Online: http://home.oise.utoronto.ca/~aresearch/artsinformed4.1.pdf.

Cancienne, M.B. (2008). From research analysis to performance: The choreographic process. In J.G. Knowles and A. Cole (Eds.), *Handbook of the arts in qualitative research: Perspectives, methodologies, examples and issues* (p. 405). Los Angeles, CA: Sage Publications.

Cole. A. (2002). *The art of research.* Toronto, ON: University of Toronto Bulletin, 12 November.

Cole, A., and Knowles, J.G. (Eds.). (2001). *Lives in context: The art of life history research.* Walnut Creek, CA: Altamira.

Cole, A., and McIntyre, M. (2003). Research as aesthetic contemplation: The role of the audience in research interpretation. *Educational Insights*, 9(1). Online: http://ccfi.educ.ubc.ca/publication/insights/v09n01/articles/cole.html.

Cole, A., and McIntyre, M. (2004). *Living and dying with dignity: The Alzheimer's project.* Online: http://home.oise.utoronto.ca/~aresearch/projects.html.

Cole, A., and McIntyre, M. (2006). *Living and dying with dignity: The Alzheimer's project*. Halifax, NS: Backalong Books. Online: http://www.ualberta.ca/~iiqm/backissues/3_2/pdf/daykin.pdf.

Denzin, N.K. (1997). *Interpretive ethnography: Ethnographic processes for the twenty-first century*. Los Angeles, CA: Sage Publications.

Eisner, E. (1991). *The enlightened eye: Qualitative inquiry and the enhancement of educational practice*. New York: Macmillan.

Eisner, E. (1993). Forms of understanding and the future of educational research. *Educational Researcher, 22*(7), 5-11.

Eisner, E. (1997). The promise and perils of alternative forms of data representation. *Educational Researcher, 26*(6), 4-10.

Ellis, C., and Bochner, A.P. (Eds.). (1996). *Composing ethnography: Alternative forms of qualitative writing*. Walnut Creek, CA: Altamira.

Finley, S. (2005). Arts-based inquiry: Performing revolutionary pedagogy. In N.K. Denzin and Y.S. Lincoln (Eds.), *The Sage handbook of qualitative research* (3rd edition) (pp. 681-94). Thousand Oaks, CA: Sage Publications.

Gladstone, B.M., Volpe, T., and Boydell, K.M. (2007). Issues encountered in a qualitative secondary analysis of help-seeking in the prodrome to psychosis. *Journal of Behavioural Health Services and Research, 34*(4), 431-42.

Glesne, C. (1997). That rare feeling: Re-presenting research through poetic transcription. *Qualitative Inquiry, 3*, 202-21.

Gray, R.E. (2000). Graduate school never prepared me for this: Reflections on the challenges of research-based theatre. *Reflective Practice, 1*(3), 377-90.

Gray, R.E. (2003). Performing on and off the stage: The place(s) of performance in arts-based approaches to qualitative inquiry. *Qualitative Inquiry, 9*, 254-67.

Gray, R.E. (2004). Performing for whom? Spotlight on the audience. In A. Cole, L. Neilsen, J.G Knowles, and T. Luciana (Eds). *Provoked by art: Theorizing arts-informed research* (pp. 238-50). Calgary, AB: Backalong Books.

Gray, R., Fitch, M., Labrecque, M., and Greenberg, M. (2003). Reactions of health professionals to a research-based theatre production. *Journal of Cancer Care, 18*(4), 223-29.

Gray, R.E., Fitch, M., Phillips, C., Labrecque, M., and Fergus, K. (2000). Managing the impact of illness: The experiences of men with prostrate cancer and their spouses. *Journal of Health Psychology, 5*, 531-48.

Gray, R.E., and Sinding, C. (2002). *Standing ovation: Performing social science research about cancer*. Walnut Creek, CA: AltaMira Press.

Gray, R.E., Sinding, C., Ivonoffski, V., Fitch, M., Hampson, A., and Greenberg, M. (2000). The use of research-based theatre in a project related to metastatic breast cancer. *Health Expectations, 3*, 137-44.

Harper, D. (1998). On the authority of the image: Visual methods at the crossroads. In Y.K. Denzin and Y.S. Lincoln (Eds.), *Collecting and interpreting qualitative materials* (pp. 130-49). Thousand Oaks, CA: Sage Publications.

Harrison, B. (2002). Seeing health and illness worlds—using visual methodologies in a sociology of health and illness: A methodological review. *Sociology of Health and Illness, 24*(6), 856-72.

Keen, S., and Todres, L. (2006). *Communicating qualitative research findings: An annotated bibliographic review of non-traditional dissemination strategies.* Bournemouth, UK: Centre for Qualitative Research at the Institute of Health and Community Studies, Bournemouth University.

Keen, S., and Todres, L. (2007). Strategies for disseminating qualitative research findings: Three exemplars. *Forum: Qualitative Social Research, 8*(3), Article 17. Online: http://www.qualitative-research.net/fqs/.

Knowles, J.G., and Cole, A.L. (Eds.) (2008). *Handbook of the arts in social science research: Methods, issues and perspectives.* Thousand Oaks, CA: Sage Publications.

Madison, D.S., and Hamera, J. (Eds.). (2006). *The SAGE handbook of performance studies.* Thousand Oaks, CA: Sage Publications.

Mason, P. (2005). Visual data in applied qualitative research: Lessons from experience. *Qualitative Research, 5*(3), 325-46.

Mienczakowski, J. (1995). The theatre of ethnography: The reconstruction of ethnography into theatre with emancipatory potential. *Qualitative Inquiry, 1*(3), 360-75.

Mienczakowski, J. (1996). An ethnographic act: The construction of consensual theatre. In C. Ellis and A.P. Bochner (Eds.), *Composing ethnography: Alternative forms of qualitative writing* (pp. 244-64). Walnut Creek, CA: AltaMira Press.

Mienczakowski, J. (1997). Theatre of change. *Research in Drama Education, 2*(2), 159-72.

Mienczakowski, J. (2003). The theatre of ethnography: The reconstruction of ethnography theatre with emancipatory potential. In N. Denzin and Y. Lincoln (Eds.), *Turning points in qualitative research: Tying knots in a handkerchief* (pp. 415-32). Thousand Oaks, CA: AltaMira Press.

Morgan, S., Rolfe, A., and Mienczakowski, J. (1993). It's funny, I've never heard voices like that before. Reporting into research performance work in schizophrenia. *Australian Journal of Mental Health Nursing, 2*(6), 266-72.

Morse, J.M. (2004). Alternative modes of representation: There are no shortcuts. *Qualitative Health Research, 14*(7), 887-88.

Mullen, C.A. (2003). Guest editor's introduction: "A self-fashioned gallery of aesthetic practice." *Qualitative Inquiry, 9*(2), 165-81.

Nisker, J., Martin, D.K., Bluhm, R., and Daar, A.S. (2006). Theatre as a public engagement tool for health-policy development. *Health Policy, 78*(2-3), 258-71.

Norris, J.R. (1997). Meaning through form: Alternative modes of knowledge representation. In J.M. Morse (Ed.), *Completing a qualitative project: Details and dialogue* (pp. 87-115). Thousand Oaks, CA: Sage Publications.

O'Connor, M. (2001). Portraits in poetry. In L. Neilsen, A.L. Cole, and J.G. Knowles (Eds.), *The art of writing inquiry.* Halifax, NS: Centre for Arts-Informed Research/Backalong Books.

Perselli, V. (2005). Re-envisioning research, re-presenting self: Putting arts media to work in the analysis and synthesis of data on "difference" and "dis/ability." *International Journal of Qualitative Studies in Education, 18*(1), 63-83.

Plummer, K. (2001). *Documents of a life: An invitation to a critical humanism.* London: Sage Publications.

Rapport, F. (2004). Introduction: Shifting sands in qualitative research. In F. Rapport (Ed.), *New qualitative methodologies in health and social care research.* New York: Routledge.

Rapport, F., Wainwright, P., and Elwyn, G. (2005). Of the edgelands: Broadening the scope of qualitative methodology. *Medical Humanities, 31,* 37-42.

Reason, P. (1988). *Human inquiry in action: Developments in new paradigm research.* London: Sage Publications.

Reason, P. (1994). *Participation in human inquiry.* London: Sage Publications.

Richardson, L. (1992). The consequences of poetic representation: Writing the other, rewriting the self. In C. Ellis and M. Flaherty (Eds.), *Investigating Subjectivity: Research on Lived Experience* (pp. 125-37). Thousand Oaks, CA: Sage Publications.

Rolfe, A., Mienczakowski, J., and Morgan, S. (1995). A dramatic experience in mental health nursing education. *Nurse Education Today, 15*(3), 224-27.

Sandelowski, M. (1998). Writing a good read: Strategies for representing qualitative data. *Research in Nursing and Health, 21*(4), 375-82.

Sandelowski, M., Trimble, F., Woodard, E.K., and Barroso, J. (2006). From synthesis to script: Transforming qualitative research findings for use in practice. *Qualitative Health Research, 16*(10), 1350-70.

Simons, H., and McCormack, B. (2007). Integrating arts-based inquiry in evaluation methodology. *Qualitative Inquiry, 13*(2), 292-311.

Smith, J.K. (2004). Crisis of representation. In M.S. Lewis-Beck, A. Bryman, and T.F. Liao (Eds.), *The Sage encyclopedia of social science research methods* (volume 3) (pp. 962-63). Thousand Oaks, CA: Sage Publications.

Sparkes, A. (2003). Review essay: Transforming qualitative data into art forms. *Qualitative Research, 3*(3), 415-20.

Thornicroft, G. (2006). *Shunned: Discrimination against people with mental illness.* Oxford: Oxford University Press.

Tilleczek, K., Cheu, H., Pong, R., Boydell, K.M., Wilson, E., and Volpe, T. (2004). *Research goes to the cinema* (paper presented at the fifth annual conference on Rural Health, Sudbury, ON).

Wainwright, P., and Rapport, F. (2007). Circles within circles—qualitative methodology and the arts: The researcher as artist (conference report). *Qualitative Social Research, 8*(3), Article 5. Online: http://www.qualitative-research.net/fqs-texte/3-07/07-3-5-e.htm.

3

Qualitative Research with Families of First Episode and Prodromal Patients

Ruth Gerson and Cheryl Corcoran

Introduction

Psychotic illness takes a toll on patients and their families, particularly the first onset of psychosis, which has been described as a "bewildering nightmare" (Gur and Johnson, 2006). Symptoms begin in adolescence and early adulthood, and are insidious and initially non-specific. Young people may not recognize the changes they are experiencing as symptoms of mental illness or may find it difficult to talk about their experiences and instead withdraw from others (Boydell, Gladstone, and Volpe, 2006; Judge, Estroff, Perkins, and Penn, 2008). They may believe that their experiences are "normal" or "just the way I was" or attribute them to stress or medical illness (Judge et al., 2008), and this explanation may be more common in minority patients (Commander, Cochrane, Sashidharan, Akilu, and Wildsmith, 1999). Although family members also may attribute the young person's behaviour and experiences to non-psychiatric etiologies (Judge et al., 2008), it is typically families who seek help for young people experiencing these emerging symptoms (de Haan, Peters, Dingemans, Wouters, and Linszen, 2002; de Haan, Linszen, Lenior, de Win, and Gorsira, 2003; de Haan, Welborn, Krikke, and Linszen, 2004; Gamble and Midence, 1994; Rose, 1996; Tuck, du Mont, Evans, and Shupe, 1997). Family members can also discourage help seeking, if they attribute the patient's behaviour to non-psychiatric etiologies (Judge et al., 2008) or they have had negative experiences with mental health treatment in the past (Compton, Kaslow, and Walker, 2004; Diala et al., 2000). Given the importance of family during the early stages of illness, understanding the experiences of families of young people with emerging psychotic symptoms can be valuable in clarifying the phenomenology of evolving illness.

Since families can play a crucial role in the path to treatment, engaging them may improve access to care for young adults experiencing new-onset psychosis. This is particularly important in light of the finding that young people with new-onset psychosis frequently go untreated for over a year (Perkins, Gu, Boteva, and Lieberman, 2005). This period of untreated psychosis is associated with significant psychosocial morbidity, poor self-esteem, and disruptions in academic and vocational achievement that are difficult to reverse (Addington, Leriger, and Addington, 2003; Tohen et al., 2000), as well as with worse long-term outcomes (Addington, Van Matrigt, and Addington, 2004; Perkins et al., 2005). Untreated psychotic symptoms can also increase the risk of suicide and victimization (Lincoln and McGorry, 1995). In addition, the cognitive deterioration seen in chronic schizophrenia appears to occur predominantly in this early period (Harrison et al., 2000). Qualitative research with families is important for understanding the behavioural manifestations of early stages of psychotic disorders and for discerning what is helpful to these young individuals and their families.

Qualitative Methods

The qualitative research methods we have employed in our studies with families were developed by Larry Davidson and his colleagues. This qualitative approach, inspired by the work of Edmund Husserl, avoids bias by prioritizing the voices of participants directly, without questionnaires or criteria, and by eliciting subjective definitions of experiences as embedded in the social context (Davidson, 1994; Fossey, Harvey, McDermott, and Davidson, 2002). Interviewers aim to approach each interview *de novo* and without bias or preconceived notions, putting out of mind the content and material of previous interviews. An open-ended approach is taken, such that the interviewers are careful not to make assumptions about the statements of their interlocutors and instead to ask clarifying questions. Interviews are unstructured in that the family member leads the dialogue. Specific topics are kept in mind by the interviewer as subjects to be queried at some point in the interview, but it is not necessarily done sequentially. In the qualitative research studies we have done with family members of both prodromal and recent-onset psychosis patients, the specific topics kept in mind included:

- what changes were perceived in the young person;
- how families responded to these changes;
- what was helpful (or not) in addressing these changes; and
- what families anticipated for the future.

Interviews were audiotaped and transcribed. Subsequently, each member of the research team individually reviewed each transcript, noting and listing themes that arose during the interviews. As with the conduct of the interviews themselves, investigators aimed to approach each transcript *de novo* in appraising themes, without considering the previous transcripts reviewed. For each transcript, the members of the research team, after independently reviewing and extracting themes from the transcript, would meet to discuss the transcript. Together, they would reach a consensus as to the themes that emerged from the transcript. This process was done for each interview/transcript.

Finally, each member of the research team independently reviewed the group of transcripts and extracted themes from each transcript in order to identify whether they sorted naturally into thematic subgroups or not. The members of the research team then reassembled the transcripts to compare independent findings and reach a consensus. Beyond the specific topics outlined earlier, other recurring themes were noted. An example in these studies is that although attribution and etiology was not specifically probed, families frequently offered explanations as to why they thought young family members had developed these problems. Of particular note in these studies, both symptomatic young individuals and family members provided informed consent. Each young person chose the family member that would be approached for the interview as someone he felt could best describe his experiences and those of his family.

Recent-Onset Psychosis: Qualitative Research with Families

In this section, we describe the findings from qualitative interviews with family members of young people with a recent onset of non-affective psychosis, which is described in greater detail in our article "Trajectory to a First Episode of Psychosis," which was published in the journal *Early Intervention in Psychiatry* (Corcoran et al., 2007). The narratives were consistent, and there was no apparent subgrouping of interviews thematically, as determined by members of the research team, both individually and in consensus meetings.

Young people were described as having previously been relatively normal but vulnerable as children and then developing clear changes in mood and behaviour in early adolescence. Family members reported having been puzzled by these changes, attributing them to a host of etiologies (commonly stress, drugs, and the "storminess" of adolescence), and they sought help initially from within social (friends, church) and family networks. Although some families initially sought help from professionals and clinicians, these attempts were largely described as being unsuccessful. Typically, treatment was finally obtained in the context of a crisis or escalation of symptoms, with emergency treatment and inpatient hospitalization, both of which were frequently involuntary. Hospitalization was perceived as traumatic, and follow-up care was described as both difficult to obtain and frustrating. Families also exhibited grief, concerns about stigma, and diminished hopes for the future.

Normal but Vulnerable as Children

Young people were typically described as having been essentially normal and happy as children, yet with some vulnerability. Some were described as sensitive, while others were shy or socially awkward: "insular," "very quiet," or showing "social immaturity" (Corcoran et al., 2007). Others had difficulty in school, with some of them struggling in speech or reading. Ostracism and teasing were also endorsed. These early "vulnerabilities," with mild deficits in social and cognitive functioning, are consistent with the subtle, non-specific abnormalities that have been described for the pre-morbid period of schizophrenia (Erlenmeyer-Kimling, 2001; Fish, Marcus, Hans, Auerbach, and Perdue, 1992; for review, see Niemi, Suvissari, Tuulio-Henriksson, and Lonnqvist, 2003). Families' lack of recognition that these vulnerabilities may presage later risk for schizophrenia is understandable, as such behaviours are non-specific and are common among many children who do not develop psychotic disorders (Olin et al., 1998). Furthermore, if these deficits represent a vulnerability to psychosis that is shared to some degree by family members, the child would not stand out as being notably different.

Insidious Changes in Mood and Behaviour in Adolescence

In many studies of this prodromal period, young people describe (and their family members confirm) symptoms of depression and irritability, social withdrawal, feelings of confusion or perplexity, suspiciousness, and a decline in functioning (Corcoran et al., 2007; Moller, 2001; Moller and Husby, 2000; Tan and Ang, 2001; Yung and McGorry, 1996). In our study, most young people were described as having had social withdrawal and anxiety: "He don't feel comfortable when people try to look in his face...he runs away from people when they come close to him." "He didn't like being around people...he was throwing up because he was nervous about all the people" (Corcoran et al., 2007). Depressive symptoms were common: "All of a sudden he didn't want to do anything. It just seemed like his life, like the doors closed and his life ended," one mother reported, while another described how her daughter stated: "I'll be alone, I don't have nothing... nothing good will happen to me" (Corcoran et al., 2007). Families also observed in the young people low motivation, sleep disturbances, little pleasure, and hopelessness, and some youth even articulated suicidal wishes. Irritability and suspiciousness of friends and family members were also reported. A changing sense of self and perplexity appears to be less frequently reported by family members than by the young people themselves (Corcoran et al., 2007; Yung and McGorry, 1996), perhaps because young people may try to hide these symptoms from family members (Boydell et al., 2006; Judge et al., 2008).

Attributions, Coping, and Help-Seeking

Families typically attribute behavioural changes to stress, adolescent turmoil, drugs, or relationship problems and only very rarely to mental illness (Compton et al., 2004; Corcoran et al., 2007; de Haan et al., 2004; Jungbauer and Angermeyer, 2002; Lincoln and McGorry, 1995; Tuck et al., 1997). Coping strategies by families appear to be motivated by these attributions and, in this sample, involved efforts at reasoning and persuasion. One mother recalled: "I yelled at him. I talked softly to him. I tried to reason with him. Nothing worked" (Corcoran et al., 2007). Many family members initially turned to friends and clergy for support and attempts at remedy, who these individuals, in turn, recommended psychiatric care: "The priest said we should take her to see a psychiatrist," "My friend told me, 'take her to the clinic'" (Corcoran et al., 2007). Often, families remember feeling that something was clearly wrong but were unsure of what to do (Corcoran et al., 2007; Singh and Grange, 2006). Understanding coping strategies is important since disparate coping strategies differentially influence help-seeking and caregiver burdens (Fortune, Smith, and Garvey, 2005; Magliano et al., 2000). Ethnic and cultural factors may also influence help seeking and coping by families (Compton et al., 2004; Runreagkulkji and Chesla, 2001; Weisman, Gomes, and Lopez, 2003).

When families in our sample did seek psychiatric help, young family members received a host of diagnoses, including substance abuse, malingering, Asperger's syndrome, depression, and "normal adolescence" (Corcoran et al., 2007), which is consistent with other studies (Singh and Grange, 2006). In addition, young people often declined help or treatment (Corcoran et al., 2007), which also follows others' findings (Czuchta and McCay, 2001). Overall, families' early attempts to seek help were experienced as stressful and confusing, which is consistent with the literature (Jungbauer and Angermeyer, 2002; Reibschleger, 1991; Wheeler, 1994; Yamashita, 1994).

The Breaking Point: Crisis and Entry into the Mental Health System

Suicidality, disorganized behaviour, and symptoms such as auditory hallucinations often prompt emergent seeking of help (Compton et al., 2004; Corcoran et al., 2007; de Haan et al., 2004). One woman in our cohort described how her daughter described feeling "not like a person," "like somebody's come and taken her out from inside her," and her daughter saying: "Mommy, I don't know what happened, the voices told me to die." One young man allegedly "started talking to himself" and "was afraid of everything," while another girl "put the phone in the sink and was washing it...I said, 'you don't wash no phone!'" Two African-American girls in our cohort were brought to treatment by police after demonstrating self-injurious or disorganized behaviour. One girl's mother described "a SWAT team" coming and was concerned that her daughter might be shot (Gerson et al., 2009). African Americans with new-onset psychosis have been found to be at increased risk of experiencing police involvement in their path to treatment (Burnett et al., 1999; Commander et al., 1999; Morgan et al., 2005a, 2005b), and, for some minority families, fears about police involvement prevent them from seeking help (Compton et al., 2004). African Americans have also been found to be more likely to fear that a person with schizophrenia will commit a violent act, which may complicate interactions with young people who may be reluctant to seek treatment (Anglin, Link, and Phelan, 2006).

Even without police involvement, hospitalization has been described as traumatic and frightening (Corcoran et al., 2007; Jungbauer and Angermeyer, 2002; Reibschleger, 1991; Wheeler, 1994). As one mother in our cohort recalled: "I will not forget when the door shut and we had to leave him in the psychiatric ward, it was a horrible feeling...I was completely in shock" (Gerson et al., 2009). Family members react to hospitalization and diagnosis with guilt and regret, but also with relief: "My putting him in the hospital was my cry for help too" (Gerson et al., 2009).

Struggling with Stigma

A first diagnosis of schizophrenia or psychosis can be terrifying for families because of the negative connotations these diagnoses carry. As one mother in our cohort remembered, "mental illness, as far as I knew, was basically untreatable" (Corcoran et al., 2007). Another mother said: "This is my whole life: dealing with mental illness." A third described feeling ashamed to tell friends that her son had mental illness, while another worried that her other children would be teased at school "because, oh, he got the brother that's the retard or whatever." Such stigma may be particularly hurtful to families as it can lead to social isolation (Lukens, Thorning, and

Lohrer, 2004; Wheeler, 1994; Wong et al., 2009), particularly for minority families (Kokanovic, Petersen, and Klimidi, 2006), and prevent help seeking (Judge et al., 2008). Feelings of guilt are also commonly associated with the stigma of mental illness (Teschinsky, 2000; Wahl and Harman, 1989) and were expressed by many family members in our cohort (Corcoran et al., 2007).

Follow-Up Care and Concerns for the Future

After the initial shock of hospitalization and diagnosis, families described facing another set of difficulties—organizing follow-up care for their loved one. While families in many countries can access specialized, youth-friendly early psychosis programs with intensive outreach, therapy, and medication, social/occupational training, and family support, such services are not widely available in the United States and were not accessible to the families in our cohort (Craig et al., 2004; O'Toole et al., 2004; Power et al., 2007). Instead, families struggled with poorly co-ordinated follow up and conflicts with third-party payers regarding coverage. Anger and frustration with the mental health system were frequently expressed (Gerson et al., 2009).

Families in our study also reported diminished expectations for the future (Corcoran et al., 2007). As one mother said, "you have expectations and hopes for your children, and if there is mental illness you just figure well that's over, pretty much." One mother described her son as "swimming against the tide" in his aspirations to attend college. Many family members worried about the longer term: "What will happen to him when we die?" "Will there be a time when I don't want to be with him anymore?" "What would happen to him?" (Corcoran et al., 2007). Some families do maintain hope for their children, wishing, for example, "that he could go get his own medication," start "talking with people, having relationships," "have a good life, find a girlfriend, a wife." Families described a desire for help in understanding psychotic illness and learning how best to care for their diagnosed family members and help them achieve their goals (Leggat, 2007; Sin, Moone, and Newell, 2007).

Defining At-Risk: Qualitative Studies of the Prodrome

Qualitative research has also been used to understand the perspectives of families of young people who have been identified as being at a heightened clinical risk for psychosis on the basis of having sub-threshold psychotic-like symptoms (Corcoran et al., 2003). Among such young people, 35 percent will develop a first episode of psychosis within 2.5 years (Cannon et al., 2008). Although retrospective studies of patients with first episode psychosis and their families shed some light on this prodromal period, concurrent descriptions of evolving symptoms by family members may improve our understanding of this phenomenology in a developmental context, which is important for developing appropriate and accessible interventions for young people and their families.

Overall: Relationship of Symptom Trajectory to Psychosis Risk

In our study of families of young people at clinically high risk for psychosis, the narratives fell thematically into two discrete groups: (1) "never normal" (that is, early and stable problems with speech, learning, motor control, and relatedness) and (2) "declining" (initially normal but vulnerable as children and then developing in adolescence clear and worrisome behavioural changes). For this second group, descriptions encompassed "a whole big turnaround—everything had changed" or, as another parent stated, "I don't even know this person. He's always been a lovable person and then this monster came out" (Corcoran et al., 2003). This second group was thematically very similar to the narratives of families of young people who had already developed a first episode of psychosis, described earlier (Corcoran et al., 2007). Not surprisingly then, the rates of conversion to psychosis were higher in this "declining" group, who had described trajectories similar to those with psychotic disorder (Corcoran et al., 2003). These findings highlight the importance of deterioration in function and the worsening of symptoms in considering psychosis risk (Moller and Husby, 2000).

The Need for Early Services

A striking theme in the narratives from both groups of prodromal patients was the profound suffering that families and patients were experiencing. Families were grappling for meaning and understanding—their attributions of symptoms included stress, drug use, spiritual crisis, normal adolescence, and genetic risk for mental illness. They described not knowing what to do, feeling "tired" and "helpless, like pounding on a brick wall" (Corcoran et al., 2003). They reported difficulties navigating the health care system and a considerable sense of burden. Clearly, these young people and their families deserve early, accessible, and affordable services, which may not only prevent or forestall psychosis onset (Gleeson, Larsen, and McGorry, 2003) but also address the significant decline in social and role function observed (Larsen et al., 2006; Larsen et al., 2007; Melle et al., 2006; Power et al., 2003).

Future Directions

Qualitative studies with families of young people in the early stages of psychotic disorder illustrate the evolution of psychotic symptoms from an essentially normal but somewhat vulnerable baseline, as well as the pain and bewilderment these families suffer. These studies complement those of young people themselves, which elucidate not only behaviours but also subjective experiences described as "torment" and "inner life dissolved" (Judge et al., 2007; Moller and Hosby, 2000). A better understanding of the phenomenology of evolving psychosis may improve the ability to illness, add to the understanding of pathophysiology in a developmental context, and lead to the development of stage-appropriate interventions that are sensitive to family, developmental, and cultural issues.

Qualitative research also focuses on the search for meaning by young people and their families. It privileges the individual's voice and experiences and is also less deficit-focused than quantitative studies based on symptom severity. For ill or at-risk youth, simple diagnosis and consequent treatment risks boxing young people into the patient role and limiting their sense of future and possibilities (Havens, 2000). It is thus important to listen closely to these young people and their families—to their experiences, needs, goals, and understanding of recovery. Only in this way can we help them emerge from the "bewildering nightmare" of early psychosis.

References

Addington, J., Leriger, E., and Addington, D. (2003). Symptom outcome one year after admission to an early psychosis program. *Canadian Journal of Psychiatry*, *48*, 204-7.

Addington, J., Van Mastrigt, S., and Addington, D. (2004). Duration of untreated psychosis: Impact on two-year outcome. *Psychological Medicine*, *34*, 277-84.

Anglin, D.M., Link, B.G., and and Phelan, J.C. (2006). Racial differences in stigmatizing attitudes toward people with mental illness. *Psychiatric Services*, *57*(6), 857-62.

Boydell, K.M., Gladstone, B.M., and Volpe, T. (2006). Understanding help seeking delay in the prodrome to first episode psychosis: A secondary analysis of the perspectives of young people. *Psychiatric Rehabilitation Journal*, *30*(1), 54-60.

Burnett, R., Mallett, R., Bhugra, D., Hutchinson, G., Der, G., and Leff, J. (1999). The first contact of patients with schizophrenia with psychiatric services: Social factors and pathways to care in a multi-ethnic population. *Psychological Medicine*, *29*, 475-83.

Cannon, T.D., Cadenhead, K., Cornblatt, B., Woods, S.W., Addington, J., Walker, E., and Heinssen, R. (2008). Prediction of psychosis in youth at high clinical risk:

A multi-site longitudinal study in North America. *Archives of General Psychiatry, 65*(1), 28-37.

Commander, M.J., Cochrane, R., Sashidharan, S.P., Akilu, F., and Wildsmith, E. (1999). Mental health care for Asian, black and white patients with non-affective psychosis: Pathways to the psychiatric hospital, in-patient and after-care. *Social Psychiatry and Psychiatric Epidemiology, 34*, 484-91.

Compton, M.T., Kaslow, N.J., and Walker, E.F. (2004). Observations on parent/family factors that may influence the duration of untreated psychosis among African American first-episode schizophrenia-spectrum patients. *Schizophrenia Research, 68*, 373-85.

Corcoran C., Davidson L., Sills-Shahar R., Nickou C., Malaspina D., and McGlashan T. (2003). A qualitative research study of the evolution of symptoms in individuals identified as prodromal to psychosis. *Psychiatric Quarterly, 35*(4), 313-32.

Corcoran, C., Gerson, R., Sills-Shahar, R., Nickou, C., McGlashan, T., Malaspina, D., and Davidson, L. (2007). Trajectory to a first episode of psychosis: A qualitative research study with families. *Early Intervention in Psychiatry, 1*, 308-15.

Craig, T.J., Garety, P., Power, P., Rahaman, N., Colbert, S., Fornells-Ambrojo, M., and Dunn, G. (2004). The Lambeth Early Onset (LEO) Team: Randomized controlled trial of the effectiveness of specialized care for early psychosis. *British Medical Journal, 329*, 1067-70.

Czuchta, D.M., and McCay, E. (2001). Help-seeking for parents of individuals experiencing a first episode of schizophrenia. *Archives of Psychiatric Nursing, 4*, 159-70.

Davidson, L. (1994). Phenomenological research in schizophrenia: From philosophical anthropology to empirical science. *Journal of Phenomenological Psychology, 25*, 104-30.

de Haan, L., Linszen, D.H., Lenior, M.E., de Win, E.D., and Gorsira, R. (2003). Duration of untreated psychosis and outcome of schizophrenia: Delay in intensive psychosocial treatment versus delay in treatment with antipsychotic medication. *Schizophrenia Bulletin, 29*(2), 341-48.

de Haan, L., Peters, B., Dingemans, P., Wouters, L., and Linszen, D. (2002). Attitudes of patients toward the first psychotic episode and the start of treatment. *Schizophrenia Bulletin, 28*(3), 431-42.

de Haan, L., Welborn, K., Krikke, M., and Linszen, D.H. (2004). Opinions of mothers on the first psychotic episode and the start of treatment of their child. *European Psychiatry, 19*(4), 226-29.

Diala, C., Muntaner, C., Walrath, C., Nickerson, K.J., LaVeist, T.A., and Leaf, P.J. (2000). Racial differences in attitudes towards professional mental health care and in the use of services. *American Journal of Orthopsychiatry, 70*(4), 455-64.

Erlenmeyer-Kimling, L. (2001). Early neurobehavioural deficits as phenotypic indicators of the schizophrenia genotype and predictors of later psychosis. *American Journal of Medical Genetics, 105*(1), 23-24.

Fish, B., Marcus, J., Hans, S.L., Auerbach, J.G., and Perdue, S. (1992). Infants at risk for schizophrenia—sequelae of a genetic neurointegrative defect: A review and replication analysis of pandysmaturation in the Jerusalem Infant Development Study. *Archives of General Psychiatry, 49*(3), 221-35.

Fortune, D.G., Smith, J.V., and Garvey, K. (2005). Perceptions of psychosis, coping, appraisals and psychological distress in the relatives of patients with schizophrenia: An exploration using self-regulation theory. *British Journal of Clinical Psychology, 44*(3), 319-31.

Fossey, E., Harvey, C., McDermott, F., and Davidson, L. (2002). Understanding and evaluating qualitative research. *Australian and New Zealand Journal of Psychiatry, 36*(6), 717-32.

Gamble, C., and Midence, K. (1994). Schizophrenia family work: Mental health nurses delivering an innovative service. *Journal of Psychosocial Nursing and Mental Health Services, 32*(10), 13-16.

Gerson, R., Davidson, L., Booty, A., McGlashan, T., Malespina, D., Pincus, H., and Corcoran, C. (2009). Families' experience with seeking treatment for recent-onset psychosis. *Psychiatric Services, 60,* 812-16.

Gleeson, J., Larsen, T.K., and McGorry, P. (2003). Psychological treatment in pre- and early psychosis. *Journal of the American Academy of Psychoanalytic and Dynamic Psychiatry, 31*(1), 229-45.

Gur, R.E., and Johnson, A.B. (2006). *If your adolescent has schizophrenia: An essential resource for parents.* Oxford: Oxford University Press.

Harrison, G., Hopper, K., Craig, T., Laska, E., Siegel, C., Wanderling, J., and Havens, L. (2000). Making a future. *American Journal of Psychotherapy, 54*(4), 477-81.

Havens, L. Making a future. *American Journal of Psychotherapy 54*(4): 477-81.

Judge, A.M., Estroff, S.E., Perkins, D.O., and Penn, D.L. (2008). Recognizing and responding to early psychosis: A qualitative analysis of individual narratives. *Psychiatric Services, 59,* 96-99.

Jungbauer, J., and Angermeyer, M.C. (2002). Living with a schizophrenic patient: A comparative study of burden as it affects parents and spouses. *Psychiatry, 65*(2), 110-23.

Kokanovic, R., Petersen, A., and Klimidi, S. (2006). "Nobody can help me...I am living through it alone": Experiences of caring for people diagnosed with mental illness in ethno-cultural and linguistic minority communities. *Journal of Immigrant and Minority Health, 8*(2), 125-35.

Larsen, T.K., Melle, I., Auestad, B., Svein, F., Haahr, U., Johannesen, J.O., and McGlashan, T. (2006). Early detection of first-episode psychosis: The effect on one-year outcome. *Schizophrenia Bulletin, 32*(4), 758-64.

Larsen, T.K., Melle, I., Friis, S., Joa, I., Johannessen, J.O., Opjordsmoen, S., and McGlashan, T.H. (2007). One-year effect of changing duration of untreated psychosis in a single catchment area (supplemental material). *British Journal of Psychiatry, 51,* 128-32.

Leggat, M.S. (2007). Minimising collateral damage: Family peer support and other strategies (supplemental material). *Medical Journal of Australia, 187*(7), 61-63.

Lincoln, C.V., and McGorry, P. (1995). Who cares? Pathways to psychiatric care for young people experiencing a first episode of psychosis. *Psychiatric Services, 46*(11), 1166-71.

Lukens, E.P., Thorning, H., and Lohrer, S.P. (2002). How siblings of those with severe mental illness perceive services and support. *Journal of Psychiatric Practice, 8*(6), 354-64.

Magliano, L., Fadden, G., Economou, M., Held, T., Xavier, M., Guarneri, M., and Maj, M. (2000). Family burden and coping strategies in schizophrenia: One-year follow-up data from the BIOMED I study. *Social Psychiatry and Psychiatric Epidemiology, 35*(3), 109-15.

Melle, I., Johannesen, J.O., Friis, S., Haahr, U., Joa, I., Larsen, T.K., and McGlashan, T. (2006). Early detection of the first episode of schizophrenia and suicidal behaviour. *American Journal of Psychiatry, 163*(5), 800-4.

Moller, P. (2001). Duration of untreated psychosis—are we ignoring the mode of initial development? An extensive naturalistic case study of phenomenal continuity in first-episode schizophrenia. *Psychopathology, 31*(4), 8-14.

Moller P., and Husby R. (2000). The initial prodrome in schizophrenia: Searching for naturalistic core dimensions of experience and behaviour. *Schizophrenia Bulletin, 26*(1), 217-32.

Morgan, C., Mallett, R., Hutchinson, G., Bagalkote, H., Morgan, K., Fearon, P., and Leff, J. (2005a). Pathways to care and ethnicity, part 1: Sample characteristics and compulsory admission (report from the AESOP study). *British Journal of Psychiatry, 186*, 281-89.

Morgan, C., Mallett, R., Hutchinson, G., Bagalkote, H., Morgan, K., Fearon, P., and Leff, J. (2005b). Pathways to care and ethnicity, part 2: Source of referral and help-seeking (report from the AESOP study. *British Journal of Psychiatry, 186*, 290-96.

Niemi, L.T., Suvissari, J.M., Tuulio-Henriksson, A., and Lonnqvist, J.K. (2003). Childhood developmental abnormalities in schizophrenia: Evidence from high-risk studies. *Schizophrenia Research, 60*(2-3), 239-58.

Olin, S.C., Mednick, S.A., Cannon, T., Jacobsen, B., Parnas, J., Schlusinger, F., and Schlusinger, H. (1998). School teacher ratings predictive of psychiatric outcome twenty-five years later (supplemental material). *British Journal of Psychiatry, 172*(33), 7-13.

O'Toole, M.S., Ohlsen, R.I., Taylor, T.M., Purvis, R., Walters, J., and Pilowsky, L.S. (2004). Treating first episode psychosis—the service users' perspective: A focus group evaluation. *Journal of Psychiatric and Mental Health Nursing, 11*, 319-26.

Perkins, D.O., Gu, H., Boteva, K., and Lieberman, J.A. (2005). Relationship between duration of untreated psychosis and outcome in first-episode schizophrenia: A critical review and meta-analysis. *American Journal of Psychiatry, 162*(10), 1785-1804.

Power, P.J., Bell, R.J., Mills, R., Herrman-Doig, T., Davern, M., Henry, H.P., and McGorry, P.D. (2003). Suicide prevention in first episode psychosis: The development of a randomized controlled trial of cognitive therapy for acutely suicidal patients with early psychosis. *Australian and New Zealand Journal of Psychiatry, 37*(4), 414-20.

Power, P., Iacoponi, E., Reynolds, N., Fisher, H., Russell, M., Garety, P., and Craig, T. (2007). The Lambeth Early Onset Crisis Assessment Team Study: General practitioner education and access to an early detection team in first-episode psychosis (supplemental material). *British Journal of Psychiatry, 51*, 133-39.

Reibschleger, J.L. (1991). Families of chronically mentally ill people: Siblings speak to social workers. *Health and Social Work, 16*(2), 94-103.

Rose, L.E. (1996). Families of psychiatric patients: A critical review and future research directions. *Archives of Psychiatric Nursing, 10*(2), 67-76.

Runreagkulkji, S., and Chesla, C. (2001). Smooth a heart with water: Thai mothers care for a child with schizophrenia. *Archives of Psychiatric Nursing, 24*(10), 1751-57.

Sin, J., Moone, N., and Newell, J. (2007). Developing services for the carers of young adults with early-onset psychosis: Implementing evidence-based practice on psycho-educational family intervention. *Journal of Psychiatric and Mental Health Nursing, 14*, 282-90.

Singh, S.P., and Grange, T. (2006). Measuring pathways to care in first-episode psychosis: A systematic review. *Schizophrenia Research, 81*(1), 75-82.

Tan, H.Y., and Ang, Y.G. (2001). First episode psychosis in the military: A comparative study of prodromal symptoms. *Australian and New Zealand Journal of Psychiatry, 35*, 512-19.

Teschinsky, U. (2000). Living with schizophrenia: The family illness experience. *Issues in Mental Health Nursing, 21*, 387-96.

Tohen M., Strakowski S.M., Zarate C., Jr, Hennen J., Stoll A.L., Suppes T., and Baldessarini, R.J. (2000). The McLean-Harvard First-Episode Project: Six-month symptomatic and functional outcome in affective and nonaffective psychosis. *Biological Psychiatry, 48*(6), 467-76.

Tuck, I., du Mont, P., Evans, G., and Shupe, J. (1997). The experience of caring for an adult child with schizophrenia. *Archives of Psychiatric Nursing, 11*(30), 118-25.

Wahl, O.F., and Harman, C.R. (1989). Family views of stigma. *Schizophrenia Bulletin, 15*(1), 131-39.

Weisman, A.G., Gomes, L.G., and Lopez, S.R. (2003). Shifting blame away from ill relatives: Latino families' reactions to schizophrenia. *Journal of Nervous and Mental Disease, 191*(9), 574-81.

Wheeler, C. (1994). The diagnosis of schizophrenia and its impact on the primary caregiver. *Nursing Praxis in New Zealand, 9*(3), 15-23.

Wong, C., Davidson, L., Anglin, D., Link, B., Gerson, R., Malaspina, D., and Corcoran, C. (2009). Stigma in families of patients in early stages of psychotic illness. *Early Intervention in Psychiatry, 3*(2), 108-15.

Yamashita, M. (1999). Newman's theory of health applied in family caregiving in Canada. *Nursing Science Quarterly, 12*(1), 73-79.

Yung, A.R., and McGorry, P.D. (1996). The initial prodrome in psychosis: Descriptive and qualitative aspects. *Australia and New Zealand Journal of Psychiatry, 30*(5), 587-99.

4

Primary Care Perspectives of First Episode Psychosis

Helen Lester

Introduction

This chapter explores the potential roles and responsibilities of the primary care team in providing care and advice for people with first episode psychosis (FEP). It starts with a discussion of the meaning of the term primary care. The chapter then focuses on the strengths and weaknesses of primary care and the role that primary care currently plays, and could play, at the point of diagnosis. The chapter concludes with a discussion of recent primary care education initiatives and some reflections on service users' views of care and international work at the "cutting edge" in this field (see Box 1).

Some Definitions of "Primary Care"

There is enormous international variation in what is meant by the term "primary care." According to the US Institute of Medicine of the National Academies (1996) primary care is the "provision of integrated, accessible healthcare services by clinicians who are accountable for addressing a

---

BOX 1: KEY POINTS

- Most primary care practitioners will see only one or two new people with FEP each year.
- While FEP is relatively rare, it is a life-changing event for the person and their family. High quality primary care at the outset offers the possibility of a less traumatic and shorter pathway into mental health services and the hope of improved longer-term outcomes.
- Primary care's recognition of early changes, clinical intuition, and ability to act on family worries are key to earlier detection.
- The primary care role may become even more important as the markers for those at highest risk become more refined.

large majority of personal health needs, developing a sustained partnership with patients, and practicing in the context of the family and community." In the United Kingdom, Martin Roland, Dave Wilkin, and Robert Boyd (1996, p. 5) suggest that primary care

> provides first-contact generalist continuing care to the great majority of health problems presented to the NHS...Primary care is, in general, located geographically close to patients' homes. It treats people in the context of their communities, and is potentially more accountable to its local community.

Primary care systems can be categorized according to whether they act as gatekeepers to specialist services (as in the United Kingdom), provide free-market services in parallel to specialist services, or function in a complex system containing both free-market and gatekeeper functionality (as in the United States); whether they are free to patients at the point of care delivery; whether they are led by doctors or non-medical personnel; and the degree to which they provide continuity of care.

Primary care in the United Kingdom has a number of unique strengths (see Box 2). It offers rapid access for routine and crisis care in a low stigma setting. It occupies an important space at the interface of users, families, communities, and professional worlds and is able to address mental, physical, and social aspects of care. Under ideal circumstances, it is also able to guarantee a cradle-to-grave doctor–patient relationship, with informational, longitudinal, and interpersonal cojntinuity of care (Saultz, 2003). Primary care is also a place of great complexity. As Iona Heath (1999, p. 565) has suggested, "uncertainty, contradiction and complexity are the stuff of general practice and the measure of much of its fascination for us."

Each day, people arrive to see their general practitioner (GP) or other member of the primary care team with coughs, colds, cancer, and depression and have, in the United Kingdom, ten minutes on average to explain their problems and negotiate a solution. This arrangement compares to

---

BOX 2: KEY STRENGTHS OF PRIMARY CARE

- offers a low stigma and accessible setting;
- enables a holistic approach to problems;
- provides informational, longitudinal, and interpersonal continuity of care;
- sees individuals in the context of their past, their social networks, and the wider community; and
- is able to deal with both the general and the particular.

the twenty-to-thirty minutes that a patient may spend in a hospital setting, to which he or she has been referred by letter to see a doctor who is an acknowledged specialist in that clinical area. In this latter case, primary care is, by way of contrast, delivered by "specialists in generalism"—by people taking an interest in whatever is of interest to the patient (Willis, 1995). Primary care, however, has developed sophisticated methodologies that are necessary for working with the uncertainty and complexity of its environment (Wilson and Holt, 2001). Decisions, for example, may be based more on intuition, experience, and knowledge of the patient's previous history than on slavish adherence to medical algorithms. This freedom should, in theory, enable GPs to rise to the challenge of diagnosing a complex condition such as FEP.

How Do People with a Psychosis Present in Primary Care?

Most GPs in the United Kingdom see only one or two new people with FEP each year. However, despite this low incidence, the role of primary care is important for a number of reasons. There is evidence that patients with a GP demonstrate a shorter duration of untreated psychosis (DUP)—that is, the time interval between the onset of psychotic symptoms and the start of anti-psychotic treatment is reduced (Skeate, Jackson, Birchwood, and Jones, 2002). GPs are frequently consulted at some point during a developing FEP and are the most common final referral agent to mental health services in the patient's pathway (Skeate et al., 2002). GP involvement is also associated with a reduced use of the *Mental Health Act* in the United Kingdom (Burnett et al., 1999).

Studies across the world of FEP have consistently found an average DUP of one to two years (McGlashen, 1999). Such delays would be unacceptable in physical illness, where a maximum two-week wait for suspected cancer referrals and two-hour "pain-to-needle" thrombolysis targets in suspected myocardial infarctions are part of standard care in the United Kingdom. It is highly likely that an association exists between a lengthy DUP and a patient's poorer outcome in FEP, particularly in regard to functional and symptomatic outcome at twelve months and in symptom reduction once treatment begins (Harrigan, McGorry, and Krstev, 2003). Long-term follow-up studies have also demonstrated that outcome at two years strongly predicts outcomes fifteen years later. Max Birchwood, Pauline Todd, and Chris Jackson (1998) argue that these observations support the concept that the early phase of psychosis represents a "critical period" in treatment, with major implications for secondary prevention of impairments and disabilities, and provide a further rationale for intervening intensively and early.

BOX 3: GP'S VIEWS ON FEP AND EIS

- 712 general practitioners from across the United Kingdom replied to the structured questionnaire in 2005 (a response rate of 24 percent).
- 47 percent felt that FEP had a favourable prognosis.
- The majority felt that the prognosis was one of a progressive decline in function.
- 9 percent felt that early detection was possible, 63 percent felt it was occasionally possible, and 19 percent felt it was not possible.
- 54 percent felt that EIS had no, or only modest, impact on patient outcomes.

Making a Diagnosis

In spite of primary care's experience in handling uncertain and complex issues, early detection of young people with a FEP is a challenge for many primary care practitioners. A recent survey in Switzerland of 1,089 GPs found that their diagnostic and treatment knowledge in FEP was inconsistent and that only one-third would continue treatment after a FEP, which is in line with international recommendations (Simon, Lauber, Ludewig, Braun-Scharm, and Umbricht, 2005). An unpublished study by the author using the same questionnaire with 712 GPs in the United Kingdom found that 95 percent of GPs had received no recent education on FEP. Most GPs also hold pessimistic views about the prognosis of FEP, its early detection, and the impact of early intervention services (EIS) (see Box 3).

Part of the challenge for primary care is that psychosis can take several months to emerge from a prodrome of non-specific psychological and social disturbances of varying intensity without clear-cut psychotic symptoms. These can include poor sleep, panic, mood changes, and social withdrawal and isolation. Positive symptoms (such as hallucinations and delusions) and negative symptoms (such as depression) are rarely volunteered spontaneously and may need to be actively sought (see Box 4).

BOX 4: SEEKING POSITIVE SYMPTOMS OF PSYCHOSIS

Questions primary care practitioners may want to ask include:

Have you felt that something odd might be going on that cannot be explained?

Have you been feeling that people are talking about you, watching you, or giving you a hard time for no reason?

Have you been feeling, seeing, or hearing things that others cannot?

Have you felt especially important in some way or that you have powers that let you do things that others cannot?

It is tempting to label some of the earlier and more vague symptoms as "normal teenage behaviour" or as a consequence of the use of cannabis. Primary care practitioners need to keep an active watching brief, to follow up missed appointments, and to take family concerns seriously. They also need a low threshold for urgently referring a young person with a suspected first episode for specialist mental health assessment.

Does GP Education Make a Difference?

There have been a small number of studies looking at the role of GP education in reducing DUP. In Singapore, the Early Psychosis Intervention Clinic program reported a lowering of the median DUP from twelve months to four months following the introduction of a public health campaign and GP education program. In Melbourne, a GP education program run by the Early Psychosis Prevention and Intervention Centre reported similar results. When patients with very long DUPs were excluded from the analysis, the DUP in the intervention sector was significantly shorter (Krstev et al., 2004). In London, United Kingdom, the Lambeth Early Onset (LEO) study evaluated the effectiveness of a GP education program and an early detection assessment team—the LEO Crisis Assessment Team—in reducing delays in accessing treatment for FEP patients (Power et al., 2007). Although the study was underpowered and the education initiative consisted of only a single twenty-five-minute session with only seventeen of the twenty-three intervention practices, they found that more intervention group GPs referred their patients directly to mental health services (86.1 percent versus 65.7 percent). However, the overall DUP was unaffected.

In Birmingham, United Kingdom, we developed an educational program in primary care to help GPs recognize and act appropriately when they see a young person with a FEP. The educational intervention is "complex" in that it comprises a number of interconnected components that are likely to interact with one another. The program was developed as the means of intervention in the REDIRECT study—a cluster randomized controlled trial (RCT) involving individuals with FEP in 108 practices in Birmingham, which aims to see if GP education leads to a change in referral patterns and DUP (Tait, Lester, Birchwood, Freemantle, and Wilson, 2005).

The REDIRECT study team, therefore, worked with a Birmingham-based EIS to develop a seventeen-minute video/CD-ROM with professional actors that included four vignettes showing how young people may present with a FEP in a primary care setting. The scenarios showed young people from different family backgrounds, some in an education setting and others at work, confused and often frightened by their symptoms. The video also contained short discussion segments between an acknowledged international expert in FEP and a GP on issues such as symptoms and signs to be alert for in FEP, suggestions for how to phrase questions, and the importance of referring all people with suspected FEP for specialist mental health assessment. A booster session, held six months after the initial educational session, aimed to reinforce knowledge and skills gained in the initial educational session and to further encourage more positive attitudes towards young people with FEP. To help facilitate a change in attitude, two users of an EIS were invited to give a short talk describing their personal experiences with FEP (Lester et al., 2005).

Following this long and complex intervention, we found that there was no difference in the numbers of referrals of people with FEP to an EIS between intervention and control practices (Lester, Birchwood, Freemantle, and Tait, in press). However, the duration of time from the first decision to seek care to the point of referral to an EIS was much shorter in patients registered in intervention practices (P = 0.002), suggesting that these cases were clearly flagged by GPs as requiring specialist care and that interfaces within secondary care had become more permeable. Analysis of pathways data also found that GPs were the most frequent first and final point of contact in the health services. The long delays we found within secondary care itself also suggest the educational messages around diagnosis and timely referral could be useful within secondary care.

The Development of EIS

Once a diagnosis is suspected or made, the young person needs to be referred on to an appropriate mental health service, ideally a service that specializes in early intervention. Early intervention in psychosis is a relatively new concept in policy terms, although claims for the benefits of intervening early in psychosis are not. In 1828, the British Metropolitan Commissioners of Lunacy made the following claim:

> Exhibiting the large proportion of cures effected in cases where patients are admitted within three months of their attacks' and the Westminster Review endorsed "the very great probability of cure in the early stages of insanity." (Scull, 1979)

However during the past two decades, the need to intervene effectively and early has become a priority in a number of countries, including the United Kingdom, Canada, New Zealand and Australia, and parts of the United States, and Scandinavia. In the United Kingdom, the lobby group Initiative to Reduce the Impact of Schizophrenia and the charity group Rethink have been at the forefront of early intervention activism, and, over a ten-year period, they have generated consistent pressure grounded in user and carer dissatisfaction with services (Rethink, 2002). Evidence from a number of countries has also demonstrated that community mental health teams (CMHTs) are less able to engage young people effectively or to provide the necessary specific treatments during the early critical period of the illness (Yung et al., 2003). RCTs have demonstrated that integrated intensive services at an early stage in the illness can lead to improved clinical outcomes, including positive and negative psychotic symptoms (Peterson et al., 2005) and lower relapse rates (Craig et al., 2004). This confluence of activism and evidence has led to the endorsement of an "early psychosis declaration" by the World Health Organization, which identified a set of expected standards of care for people with FEP (see the discussion later this chapter).

In the United Kingdom in 2000, a major policy reform entitled the National Plan for the National Health Services stated that "fifty early intervention teams will be established by 2004 so that...all young people who experience a first episode of psychosis, such as schizophrenia will receive the early and intensive support they need" (Department of Health, 2001, p. 19). This statement was supported by a number of policy implementation guides, which provided technical detail and practical strategies for the newly funded services that were to follow as well as for a National Early Intervention Programme to oversee the development of the new services (Department of Health 2001; Department of Health, 2002).

By March 2005, an audit by the National Early Intervention Programme found that eighty-six new "functionalized" EIS had been implemented and were able to deliver services to approximately one-third of the population in the United Kingdom (Pinfold, Smith and Shiers, 2007). For primary care practitioners in the United Kingdom, however, this development means that the most common pathway into services when they suspect a young person of having a FEP is still to refer them to existing CMHTs.

Recent Primary Care Policy Initiatives

In Autumn 2007, guidance to help front-line practitioners achieve earlier diagnosis of psychosis in young people was launched by the Royal College of General Practitioners and the Royal College of Psychiatrists in the United Kingdom. The guidance was designed following a report commissioned by the National Institute for Mental Health in England, which highlights the growing evidence base that early symptom recognition can reduce the progression to psychosis. The advice for GPs lists key symptoms, which may signal the onset of psychosis, and aims to create a smoother pathway between primary care practitioners and mental health specialists to ensure

TABLE 1: EARLY PSYCHOSIS DECLARATION RELATING TO PRIMARY CARE

EARLY PSYCHOSIS DECLARATION	RELATING TO PRIMARY CARE
Comprehensive program	**Measured outcome**
• Improve access and engagement • Walk-in responsive services usually provided in primary care settings should be equipped to deal effectively with early psychosis • Service interfaces should be designed to support quicker and more effective engagements of young people	• The mean DUP from the onset of psychosis should be less than three months • The use of involuntary treatments in the first engagement should be less than 25 percent • Effective treatment should be provided after no more than three attempts to seek help
• Practitioner training • All primary care sites should be equipped to deal effectively with early psychosis • Continued professional development should be supported for all specialist staff working with young people. with psychosis	• Recognition, care, and treatment of young people with psychosis should be a routine part of training curricula of all primary care and social care practitioners • Specific early intervention training programs should be resourced and evaluated

early detection and provide vital support for young people with psychosis and their families. The pivotal role of primary care in care pathways is also highlighted in the Early Psychosis Declaration (Betolote and McGorry, 2005) (see Table 1).

What Do Service Users Think?

From the service users' perspectives, there has been very little written about views on primary care at the point of an FEP. Previous work has highlighted a perceived lack of information and explanation for patients about diagnosis and treatment (Bailey, 1997), overuse of medication and a delay in obtaining a diagnosis (Rogers and Pilgrim, 1993), and barriers created by stigmatized attitudes (Kai and Crosland, 2001). More recently, focus groups with service users who have been living with a psychosis for an average of eight years, GPs, and practice nurses have provided further insights into this area of care (Lester, Tritter, and Sorohan, 2005) (see Box 5).

An important "bottom line" here is that although GPs may feel that lack of knowledge inhibits greater involvement in care, patients with psychosis value a continuity of care, good listening skills, advocacy, and a willingness to learn more than just a specific knowledge about mental health. A GP who knows them, listens to them, and can access help for mental health problems when required would be viewed by almost all patients as "good enough."

BOX 5: PROVIDING "GOOD ENOUGH" PRIMARY CARE

- Most service users in the study viewed primary care as the "cornerstone" of their physical and mental health care.
- Service users and health professionals agreed that the latter had a responsibility to continue prescribing drugs started in secondary care, monitor side effects, and tackle physical health issues. Both groups recognized, however, that it was sometimes difficult to present with, or diagnose, physical complaints once a mental health disorder had been diagnosed. Some GPs suggested that this issue was related to difficulties in communicating effectively with people with serious mental illness.
- Most health professionals perceived the mental health care of people with serious mental illness as being too specialized for routine primary care and felt they lacked sufficient skills and knowledge.
- All participants felt that interpersonal and longitudinal continuity was vital for good quality care. However, most health professionals felt continuity was threatened by other national primary care policies.
- Service users felt that continuity helped to ensure accurate diagnosis, particularly at times of mental health crisis; prevented the retelling of painful stories; enabled trust to develop that in turn facilitated discussions of treatment options; and, above all, allowed patients and health professionals to understand each other as people.
- Most service users favoured seeing the same GP for their physical and mental health needs, preferring a continuous doctor-patient relationship and a positive attitude and willingness to learn, rather than the opportunity to consult a different GP with special expertise in mental health.
- Most service users knew that their GP had little formal training in mental health and did not expect expert advice from primary care professionals.

There are definitely challenges ahead for primary care as young people who have experienced an episode of psychosis are discharged from EIS into primary care. At the moment in the United Kingdom, approximately 50 percent of people who have experienced an FEP have no formal mental health follow-up at discharge and so will be seen and treated for their physical and mental health problems by primary care practitioners. These individuals will have much to live up to! Semi-structured interviews with thirty-two service users, purposively sampled on age, gender, and ethnicity from eleven of the twelve active EIS in the West Midlands region of England found that almost all had been anxious at the prospect of being referred to a mental health service but described the reality of engaging with them as very positive. The EIS were staffed by people who were "consistent," "knew what they were doing," "cared," "weren't pushy but listened," and were "very helpful and gave lots of information." The EIS had helped by giving them information that addressed their stereotypes, reduced their fears about the future, and increased their self confidence so they were more able to talk to friends and employers about their illness (Lester et al., 2009). However, most of the focus, certainly in UK services and commissioning bodies has been on the "front end," with far less attention being paid to ongoing care and follow-up services. However, we know that this group of young people are at a higher risk than those individuals suffering from cardiovascular problems at an earlier age (Saha, Chant, and McGrath, 2007) and are also at risk of relapse and suicide. Therefore, engaged generalist practitioners who are aware of the issues are vital. It remains to be seen, however, if primary care practitioners can recognize and step up to this challenge.

Where Next?

There are a number of cutting-edge issues in terms of primary health care and psychosis nationally and internationally, particularly with respect to the role of primary care in detecting young people with "at risk mental states" (ARMS). As the markers for those individuals at highest risk become more refined, there is hope that very early detection and intervention could reduce the progression to psychosis. Several studies are currently testing whether cognitive behavioural therapy (CBT) and/or low-dose antipsychotic medication offered to individuals at ultrahigh risk of psychosis can reduce the risk of subsequent psychosis as well as ameliorate prodromal symptoms. Two such trials have already reported promising results. The Promoting Healthy Ageing with Cognitive Exercise (PACE) study in Melbourne has shown a reduction in the risk of FEP from 35 percent to 10 percent while patients are being treated with low-dose atypical antipsychotics and CBT, but the benefits disappeared when the treatment was withdrawn (McGorry et al., 2002). Anthony Morrison and his colleagues (2004) have demonstrated almost the same lowered conversion rate to psychosis (that is, 12 percent) with CBT alone in a similar group of patients. So far, however, these studies have been conducted in relatively small samples of people at a high risk of psychosis, who are willing to seek help, and who are in a research setting. It remains to be seen if the findings can be translated into a real world intervention that is widely available to individuals with ARMS. Nevertheless, for primary care, the implications of these studies are considerable. They could, for example, shift the focus towards primary care recognition and the necessity to flag individuals with key "at-risk" indicators and point patients towards a different access route that involves a youth-oriented specialist assessment and psychological treatment service.

Conclusions

Early intervention is everyone's business. The incidence of FEP may be low at an individual practice level, but the consequences for the person and their family can be devastating and long lasting. We know GPs are key pathway players, typically prompted by help seeking that is initiated by families. Furthermore, the GP role may become even more important as the markers for those individuals at highest risk (the so-called ARMS) become more refined. Research is increasingly showing that very early detection and intervention may reduce the progression towards psychosis, and we now must await evidence for whether these findings can be translated into practical interventions that are widely available.

Primary care practitioners need easy access to specialist advice and assessment for individuals with suspected FEP, who could in turn be engaged within a less stigmatizing and more easily accessible environment. EIS also have a role to play in helping to address GP knowledge gaps and attitudes towards young people with FEP. When such levels of partnership are achieved, care pathways may be shorter and less traumatic, and the Early Psychosis Declaration could become an interesting historical footnote.

References

Bailey, D. (1997). What is the way forward for a user-led approach to the delivery of mental health services in primary care? *Journal of Mental Health*, 6, 101-5.

Betolote, J., and McGorry, P. (2005) Early intervention and recovery for young people with early psychosis: Consensus statement (supplemental material). *British Journal of Psychiatry*, 187, 116-19.

Birchwood, M., Todd, P., and Jackson, C. (1998) Early intervention in psychosis: The critical period hypothesis (supplemental material). *British Journal of Psychiatry*, 172(33), 53-59.

Burnett, R., Mallett., R., Bhugra, G., Hutchinson, G., Der, G., and Leff, J. (1999). The first contact of patients with schizophrenia with psychiatric services: Social factors and pathways to care in multi-ethnic population. *Psychological Medicine*, 29, 475-83.

Craig, T., Garety, P., Power, P., Rahaman, N., Colbert, S., Fornell-Ambrojo, M., and Dunn, G. (2004). The Lambeth Early Onset (LEO) Team: Randomised controlled trial of the effectiveness of specialised care for early psychosis. *British Medical Journal*, 329, 1067-71.

Department of Health (United Kingdom). (2001). *The Mental Health Policy Implementation Guide*. Online: http://www.dh.gov.uk/en/Publicationsandstatistics/ Publications/PublicationsPolicyAndGuidance/DH_4009350.

Department of Health (United Kingdom). (2002). *Improvement, expansion and reform: The next three years—priorities and planning framework 2003–2006*. Online: http://www.dh.gov.uk/en/Publicationsandstatistics/ Publications/ PublicationsPolicyAndGuidance/DH_4008430.

Harrigan, S.M., McGorry, P.D., and Krstev, H. (2003). Does treatment delay in first episode psychosis really matter? *Psychological Medicine*, 33, 97-110.

Heath, I. (1999). Uncertain clarity: Contradiction, meaning and hope. *British Journal of General Practice, 49,* 651-57.

Institute of Medicine of the National Academies. (1996). *Primary care: America's health in a new era* (consensus report). Online: http://www.iom.edu/Reports/1996/Primary-Care-Americas-Health-in-a-New-Era.aspx.

Kai, J., and Crosland, A. (2001). Perspectives of people with enduring mental ill health from a community-based qualitative study. *British Journal of General Practice, 51,* 730-37.

Krstev, H., Carbone, S., Harrigan, S., Curry, C., Elkins, K., and McGorry, P.D. (2004). Early intervention in first-episode psychosis: The impact of a community development campaign. *Social Psychiatry and Psychiatric Epidemiology, 39,* 711-19.

Lester H.E., Birchwood, M., Bryan, S., England, E., Rogers, H., and Sirvastava, N. (2009). Development and implementation of early intervention services for young people with psychosis: A case study. *British Journal of Psychiatry, 194*(5), 446-50.

Lester H.E., Birchwood, M., Freemantle, N., and Tait, L. (in press). REDIRECT: A randomised controlled trial to evaluate the role of education in reducing duration of untreated psychosis in primary care. *British Journal of General Practice.*

Lester, H.E., Tait, L., Khera, A., Birchwood, M., Freemantle, N., and Patterson, P. (2005). The development and evaluation of an educational intervention on first episode psychosis for primary care. *Medical Education, 39,* 1006-14.

Lester, H. E., Tritter, J.Q., and Sorohan, H. (2005) Patients' and health professionals' views on primary care for people with serious mental illness: Focus group study. British Medical Journal, 330, 1122-27.

McGlashan, T.M. (1999). Duration of untreated psychosis in first episode schizophrenia: Marker or determinant of course. *Biological Psychiatry, 46,* 899-907.

McGorry, P., Yung, A.R., Phillips, L.J., Yuen, H.P., Francey, S., Cosgrave, M., and Jackson, H. (2002). Randomized controlled trial of interventions designed to reduce the risk of progression to first-episode psychosis in a clinical sample with subthreshold symptoms. *Archives General Psychiatry, 59,* 921-28.

Morrison, A.P., French, P., Walford, L., Lewis, S.W., Kilcommons, A., Green, J., and Bentall, R. (2004). Cognitive therapy for the prevention of psychosis in people at ultra-high risk: Randomized controlled trial. *British Journal of Psychiatry, 185,* 291-97.

Petersen, L., Nordentoft, M., Jeppensen, P., Thorup, A., Christensen, T.O., Krarup, G., Dahstrom, J., Haastrup, B., and Jorgensen, P. (2005). Improving one-year outcome in first-episode psychosis (supplemental material). *British Journal of Psychiatry, 187,* 90-103.

Pinfold, V., Smith, J., and Shiers, D. (2007). Audit of early intervention in psychosis service development in England in 2005. *Psychiatric Bulletin, 31,* 7-10.

Power, P., Iacoponi, E., Reynolds, N., Fisher, H., Russell, M., Garety, P., and Craig, T. (2007). The LEO crisis assessment team study: General practitioners education and access to an early detection team in first episode psychosis (supplemental material). *British Journal of Psychiatry, 191*, 133-39.

Rethink. (2002). *Reaching people early: A status report received by people with severe mental illness and their informal carers.* London: Rethink.

Rogers, A., and Pilgrim, D. (1993). *Experiencing psychiatry: Users' views of services.* London: Macmillan Press.

Roland, M., Wilkin, D., and Boyd, R. (1996). Rationale for moving towards a primary care-led NHS. In National Primary Care Research and Development Centre (Ed.), *What is the future for a primary care?* (pp. 5-12). Oxford: Radcliffe Medical Press.

Saha S., Chant D., and McGrath J. (2007). A systematic review of mortality in schizophrenia: Is the differential mortality gap worsening over time? *Archives of General Psychiatry, 64*, 1123-31.

Saultz, J.W. (2003) Defining and measuring interpersonal care. *Annals of Family Medicine, 3*, 134-44.

Scull, A.T. (1979) *Museums of madness: The social organization of insanity in nineteenth-century England.* New York: St. Martin's Press.

Simon, A., Lauber, C., Ludewig, K., Braun-Scharm, H., and Umbricht, D.S. (2005). General practitioners and schizophrenia: Results from a Swiss survey. *British Journal of Psychiatry, 187*, 274-81.

Skeate, A., Jackson, C., Birchwood, M., and Jones, C. (2002). Duration of untreated psychosis and pathways to care in first-episode psychosis (supplemental material). *British Journal of Psychiatry, 181*, 73-77.

Tait, L., Lester, H.E., Birchwood, M., Freemantle, N., and Wilson, S. (2005). Design of the Birmingham early detection in untreated psychosis trial (REDIRECT): Cluster randomised controlled trial of general practitioner education in detection of first episode psychosis. *BMC Health Services Research, 5*, 19.

Willis, J. (1995). *The paradox of progress.* Abingdon, UK: Radcliffe Medical Press.

Wilson, T., and Holt, T. (2001). Complexity science: Complexity and clinical care. *British Medical Journal, 323*(7314), 685-88.

Yung, A.R., Phillips, L.J., Yuen, H.P., Francey, S.M., Hallgren, M., and McGorry, P.D. (2003). Psychosis prediction: Twelve-month follow up of a high-risk ("prodromal") group. *Schizophrenia Research, 60*, 21-32.

Suggested Further Reading

Lester, H. (2001). Ten-minute consultation: First episode psychosis. *British Medical Journal, 323*, 1408.

Shiers, D., Lester, H. (2004). Early intervention for first episode psychosis. *British Medical Journal, 328*, 1451–52.

Useful Internet Addresses
Initiative to Reduce the Impact of Schizophrenia (IRIS): http://www.iris initiative.org.uk/

The Early Intervention in Psychosis IRIS network supports the promotion of EI in psychosis. Its other aims are to encourage the development of services that are non-stigmatizing and appropriate to the needs of young people in the early stage of illness; to reduce the impact of psychosis on young people; and to encourage and develop better mental health promotion schemes to highlight the benefits of early intervention to key audiences.

Psychosis Sucks, a program of the Fraser Health Early Intervention (EPI) Program: http://www.psychosissucks.ca/epi/aboutepi.cfm

A Canadian website that promotes early detection, educates about psychosis, and provides direction for seeking help.

Early Psychosis Prevention and Intervention Clinic (EPPIC), http://www .eppic.org.au/

An Austrian site that describes the work of the EPPIC group and includes information on a range of resources such as training manuals, videos, DVDs.

5

Hearing Echoes: Image Identification and the Clinicians' (Learning) Experience with Early Intervention

Joan McIlwrick

What knowledge and mystery are present in our patients and in our encounters, and are we able to learn from them? (Killackey, Yung, and McGorry, 2007)

Introduction

What can we learn about a person in the early stages of a psychotic illness if we see the experience from the perspective of the clinicians that care for these patients? What do clinicians learn about themselves when they work alongside a person with a developing psychotic disorder? Are these questions worth exploring, and, if so, how do we explore them? Moreover, how can these stories be told? These were the ideas I was considering in October 2007 during the inaugural meeting of the International Early Psychosis Qualitative Research Consortium in Toronto, where I was seated at the same table as several veteran early interventionists. Hearing the passionate opinions, stories, and occasional debates from this international group of researchers and clinicians made me reflect upon the types of experiences that shape our professional lives. Of particular interest to me was, and is, the impact that people experiencing the early stages of psychosis have upon the clinicians they encounter.

My interest in the clinician experience has developed over the past ten years. My professional path has led me to meet two people with early stage psychosis at pivotal moments in my training, and the impact of these encounters has clearly influenced the work I continue to do. When I was a third-year medical student, seriously considering quitting medical school, it was because a young woman with a psychotic disorder volunteered her time and personal story with my group of clinical skills students that I became interested in a career in psychiatry. Although there were many reasons why I became a psychiatrist, it was ultimately because Mary shared her story with a group of medical students that I started down this road.

If Mary was the start of my work in psychiatry, then Ray is the reason I believe in early intervention. Ray was a man I met midway through my residency, while he was in what I now understand to be the psychosis prodrome. For various reasons, he never received early intervention, and I encountered him over several years of my residency, usually when he appeared in the emergency room when I was on call. His condition deteriorated to the point of homelessness over those years, and he will always be a reminder to me of the importance of early intervention for young people with mental illness.

Neither Mary nor Ray ever knew the impact they had on my development as a clinician, primarily because it took years before I understood the extent of the impact for myself. In an era of "Code Burgundy" (the term used to define too many patients and not enough hospital beds), overcrowding in the emergency room (Canadian Association of Emergency Physicians (CAEP), 2007), overcapacity on the units, long wait-lists in the clinics, and other demands on the time and attention of clinicians, there is little time for self-reflection on what we learn from our patients, both about their experiences and about our own. The purpose of this chapter is to provide you with the opportunity to experience reflections from residents, psychiatrists, and nurses on their work alongside people with early stage psychosis.

How Does This Chapter Fit into the Current Early Psychosis Landscape?

Early intervention for psychotic disorders is said to date back 200-300 years, starting in the 1700s when "lunatics" were relabelled as "patients." Over time, people with psychotic illnesses were moved from "asylum cells" to "curable" wards where they received treatment and were no longer on display as entertainment to the fee-paying public (Reame, 2002). Generally, early intervention in psychosis refers to the movement, started in the early 1990s, that includes researchers, patients, clinicians, caregivers, and policy makers, who were all focused on the early identification and treatment of people with psychotic disorders. A recent summary of the early psychosis field comprises key issues such as focusing primarily on matters related to the duration of untreated illness as well as the economics, timing, and ethics of early intervention (Killackey, Yung, and McGorry, 2007). Understandably, the focus of early intervention work to date has used quantitative methods and focused primarily on topics related to psychosis as a biological syndrome, with measurable psychosocial consequences.

Almost nothing is known about the clinician experience in early intervention. Work has been done using quantitative methods to measure clinician reaction to a specific diagnosis (no correlation was found between the diagnosis and the way in which staff felt towards the patients) (Holmqvist, 1998). There is more to the story than can be told with measures and scales, and, thus, a qualitative exploration of this topic can provide an alternative perspective. There is certainly an interest within the lay public for stories written from the doctor's perspective about doctor–patient experiences, if the 2007 Giller Prize award to a physician for his collection of stories based on his experience with patients is any indication (Lam, 2006).

The following pages will reveal the clinician's experience with early intervention from the clinician's own words. Two different groups will be telling their stories. One group consists of a team of three relatively experienced early interventionists (a psychiatrist, a nurse, and a family worker with forty-five years of combined experience), who share their thoughts about starting an ultra-high-risk/prodrome clinic. In addition to the veteran early interventionist stories are accounts from psychiatry residents (doctors in specialty training to become psychiatrists), who share their encounters with patients in crisis in the emergency department, making these residents "apprentice early interventionists" by necessity. Although this collection of people appears to be quite different in terms of background and practice, what they do have in common is the fact that they are all meeting people in the early stages of psychosis and that this meeting has an impact.

The original reason for collecting the thoughts of the veteran group was to document their experiences of developing a new clinic in the relatively uncharted waters of "ultra-high risk." The stories from the psychiatry residents were collected as part of a larger study of the resident experience while they were on call in the emergency room. Over the two years that these data were being collected as part of separate projects, it became apparent that there were similarities in the veteran and resident clinician experiences in their encounters with early stage psychosis patients. The possible explanation for these similarities is discussed at the end of this chapter, as are the implications for the larger early intervention field.

We Learn from Our Patients

The overarching theme that becomes clear in a review of the stories from both the veteran and the resident stories is that these clinicians have learned from their encounters with patients of early stage psychosis. This does not come as a surprise, given that clinical training, be it in nursing, medicine, or most other areas of health care, is patient-centred. It is important to note, however, that the lessons that we learn from patients can be categorized in two ways: the stated curriculum and the hidden curriculum (Lempp and Seale, 2004). In medical training, for example, there are the lessons taught according to the defined (stated) medical school or residency curriculum (Brodkey, Van Zant, and Sieries, 1997; Royal College of Physicians and Surgeons of Canada (RCPSC), 2007a). These lessons are derived from topics that follow part of a long-standing tradition (such as the standard approach to collecting medical history) and part of the trend of the day (such as how to use a palm-pilot in everyday practice). Whatever the reason that a topic is found on a medical school or residency curriculum, the topic list is strictly defined and enforced by accreditation standards and committees (RCPSC, 2007b). The success by which students learn their lessons are closely tracked and studied by medical educators. A great deal, therefore, is known about the lessons that we think we are teaching clinicians.

There is very little in the academic and scientific literature that explores the lessons that doctors learn from their ordinary, and extraordinary, interactions with patients. This information is referred to as "hidden curriculum learning" (Lempp and Seale, 2004). The concept refers to lessons learned when we do not even know it is happening—lessons that are never listed on an educational curriculum. Some of these lessons are positive— for example, when a student observes a preceptor spending extra time with a person in distress, even though the rest of the clinic is going to run late, she learns that such behaviour can be acceptable. Some of these lessons are negative though—for example, a student observing a preceptor talking about a patient in an elevator, which is in violation of confidentiality rules, concludes, erroneously, that such behaviour is acceptable. While the academic literature is only beginning to explore hidden curriculum learning, the lay public has had access to health care provider accounts of lessons learned from "war stories" for many years (Pekkanen, 1988). Jeffrey Borkan and William Miller (1999) offer a beautiful description of the rise and fall of storytelling in medicine, noting that in the age of "technomedicine" the average clinician allows a patient only eighteen seconds of narrative prior to interrupting and reverting back to a focus on doctor-oriented disease topics, which reduces the patient experience to a checklist of symptoms rather than a richly detailed story from which we can learn.

A review of a sample of stated learning objectives for physician training in early psychosis reveals a standard list of topics that a physician is expected to know in the management of a patient with psychosis (Department of Psychiatry, University of Calgary, n.d.). A review of what clinicians tell us they learn about patients paints a more complex picture. One resident explains the difference between learning about what is formally taught (that is, in lectures about psychosis) and what is learned from a reflection upon the experience in the emergency room through conversations with the patients themselves:

I think sometimes the best learning you can get from patients is after the fact. We learn about the acute presentation of psychosis, but talking to them, once they're stabilized, about what that was like for them and what they were experiencing and how they experienced the nursing staff and the security and you. I think that's huge. (Resident)

Emergency rooms are generally staffed by resident physicians. When thinking of early intervention for psychosis, what usually comes to mind are the organized services, outpatient clinics, and philosophical movement designed to provide care to patients in the early stages of psychotic disorders. It may not be immediately obvious that the front-line physicians-in-training, working on call in the emergency departments are also providing early intervention for psychotic patients in crisis. As this resident points out,

[working in the ER] gives you a good appreciation for people presenting for the first time, or what they look like when they are first arriving for care. Whereas, when you are working in other areas, you do not have an idea of exactly how they come into the system, or what they look like, because they have been assessed by someone else, or have already been partially treated. It gives you tools to use when people are presenting in distress. (Resident)

The emergency room is an environment notorious for the tension and demands placed upon trainees (Brasch and Ferencz, 1999). Accreditation bodies protect resident physicians against the imbalances between education and service (RCPSC, 2007b). Nowhere are residents more vigilant about education-to-service imbalances than in the emergency room. It is because of this vigilance that resident responses about what they learn in the emergency room are particularly valid—they think about it frequently. It is in the emergency room that the resident is most likely to encounter the first episode patient as he or she enters the mental health system:

When a psychotic patient presents, most often times, that's the textbook instances, when you're on-call and see someone like that. Probably the strongest memories that a lot of us have of different patients or different situations would be in the emergency room. (Resident)

Although it is the fundamental job of the resident to learn and train, clinicians-in-practice are also learning on an ongoing basis through their daily work with patients. As this veteran early interventionist points out when discussing the experience of establishing an ultra-high-risk/prodrome clinic:

> This [starting a prodrome clinic] has been so challenging, in part because of the diagnostic and management challenges. I feel intellectually tested each day, and I think there has been a steep learning curve that has surprised me. The experience that I brought with me from the early psychosis work has not translated directly to the prodrome work, and I have had to learn new skills and concepts very quickly. (Veteran)

The next section further details the lessons that resident and veteran clinicians say they have learned from their work with people in the early stages of psychosis.

What Do We Learn from Our Work with Patients?

We Learn about Challenges Dealing with "the System"

A review of the academic literature related to early psychosis reveals minimal information on the patient perspective of the mental health system. However, the studies that have been published suggest that patients and families struggle with their entry into mental health care services, feeling as though they are "invisible and silent partners in care" and "undervalued by mental health services" (Sin, Moore, and Wellman, 2005, p. 589). This sentiment is echoed in the findings of Barbara Schneider and Colin McDonald (2008), in which one patient claims that patients themselves are in fact people and not just another thing to manage.

The resident and veteran clinicians acknowledge that the patient with early stage psychosis encounters challenges with "the system." This resident ponders the importance of being aware of patient challenges, asking about these experiences and trying to learn from them:

> I think there's a ton to learn from patients. As they enter the system, they have a variety of experiences, some good, some not so good, and so if you're sort of open to hearing about their experiences, I think, there's a lot to be learned there... even just being able to ask patients about what they've found helpful in the past and what they haven't found helpful is very useful for our learning. (Resident)

The idea of learning about the patient experience is similarly echoed by veteran early interventionists as well:

I think the entry into this system must be bewildering for patients, on such a basic level. I remember when I first started working at this huge hospital, how hard it was for me to find my way around for the first several months, all the paperwork I had to do to get my paycheque and parking and so on. When a patient arrives for an appointment now, flustered because he or she is late, and got lost, and couldn't find my office or the lab, I feel badly about it. How difficult must this process be for someone who is beginning to experience cognitive decline, especially when the deficits are very early? (Veteran)

Some people might find it distasteful that a clinician is so open about the idea of benefiting from the discomfort and distress of a patient. Others would say it is a refreshing change and possibly represents a shift in the medical culture—namely that a physician is less interested in reducing the patient to a symptom checklist and more interested in how one person's experience might benefit the experience for the next. The fact that the early stage psychosis patient can still teach the clinician is an example of a valuable hidden curriculum lesson.

We Learn What It Is Like to Deal with Uncertainty

Doctors have long been portrayed as being unaccustomed to not knowing. Medical school and residency training, with the "pass–fail" system of single, correct-answer multiple choice exam questions, teaches physicians that the correct answer can always be known (another example of a hidden curriculum lesson). Clinicians working with patients in the early stages of psychosis learn that the opposite is usually true. They learn how to deal with uncertainty:

Sometimes, the story you get from the family may be a lot different than the story you're getting from the patient. You may start off thinking about one diagnosis, and then you're wondering: "Is this something acutely psychotic here?" (Resident)

In the emergency room, the resident must make rapid diagnostic and management decisions that may lead to significant consequences for the patient, such as the temporary removal of the right to freedom (possible, according to most jurisdictional mental health acts). The resident, therefore, must know as much as possible what is going on with a patient.

However, residents working with families and patients in the emergency room learn that the first presentation is not always clear-cut, particularly if a patient is presenting in the prodrome or very early stages of psychosis. Such lessons are not necessarily taught in lectures or in the *Diagnostic and Statistical Manual of Mental Disorders* (American Psychiatric Association, 2000), which tells trainees that psychosis generally equals hallucinations and delusions. The first episode patient, therefore, teaches trainees that

> *the sicker the patient, the easier it is to make decisions. Whereas, the less sick they seem to appear, the harder it is, which is so different from other conditions. (Resident)*

The level of uncertainty described by the residents was not fundamentally different than the uncertainty revealed by the veteran team working with the prodrome patient:

> *The ones who show up and want treatment—what are you going to do with them? The literature is still talking about the ethics of treating the prodrome, and there is very little guidance for a clinician who has made the decision to treat. The situation is even more complex when using a psychotropic medication on a minor patient, with a condition that is not even defined in the DSM-IV. It feels like very shaky ground. (Veteran)*

The veteran team, like the residents, describe struggling with how to make the decision to diagnose and manage patients in the early stages of psychosis. Interestingly, both groups also identified that the struggles are not limited to the matter of medication or hospitalization. In other words, the patient with early stage psychosis teaches clinicians that there is more to patient care than can be found on the prescription pad.

We Learn That Patients Need More Than Just a Prescription

The "bio-psychosocial framework" is the current cornerstone of the mental health care curriculum (Dowling and Engel, 2005). However, the lessons hung on the bio-psychosocial skeleton are sometimes biased in favour of biology. An example of such a biological bias can be found in a recent review of the majority of the key topics in early psychosis intervention. With the focus on how to choose an antipsychotic medication, how to manage metabolic syndrome, and when to offer interventions to patients, psychosocial elements appear to be less in focus predominant in academic literature and, therefore, not as highly emphasized in health care curricula.

It is not until clinicians encounter actual patients that the hidden curriculum teaches them what is needed in the care of the patient, as the following excerpts reveal:

> One thing really struck me was when I was trying to advocate for a patient. We decided we were going to send her home and I was trying to negotiate to get a taxi chit for this woman and the ER staff said: "We're not here just to give handouts." It's interesting because you do learn a lot about your role as a mental health advocate and you get a sense through those experiences as to how the medical system can butt up and prevent progress for people who have certain deficits. So, I've definitely felt that way, that I was in the role of advocate and that somehow the rest of the emergency environment was against me, in that. (Resident)

This veteran interventionist described similar lessons learned in terms of understanding the value of providing care other than medication for the early stage psychosis patient. In this excerpt, the clinician explains how she learned that trying to "fix" problems with medication was less useful than supporting the patients with education and reassurance:

> I needed to change my thinking to realize that it was helping to educate, to reassure. Patients would come in and describe negative and cognitive symptoms, and I was trying to fix that for them. I learned from the case manager who would educate patients, and tell them, that is part of the illness, which is just the way it is. It was as though I needed to give medication for myself, but the patients did OK with education and an understanding. (Veteran)

Similarly, this interventionist described coming to the realization that "part of the job" is helping patients to cope with their illness through an acceptance of the circumstances rather than trying to find a treatment in terms of a cure:

> Part of our job is to help the person live with the circumstance, not necessarily to cure it, and to me, from a nursing perspective, that is what medicine is. To me, health is not having illness, it is growing and progressing with the circumstance. (Veteran)

We Learn to Conceptualize the Illness Differently
Of course, no clinician can ever proclaim to fully understand the patient experience, save for the clinicians who have become patients themselves.

However, the clinicians who pay attention to the time they spend with their patients and to the stories they hear from their patients learn to think differently about what their patients are facing. In the case of the veteran early interventionists working for the first time with prodrome patients, they learned that a shift in their understanding of the illness that they thought they understood needed to be reframed:

> When I started this clinic, I had the misconception that ultra-high-risk patients were healthy people who were simply at "high risk." I now realize they are not healthy, because they are declining at school, or work, or have a subjective sense of being unwell. (Veteran)

As a result, the clinicians learned to reformat their entire approach to the patient:

> Because of my experience in the prodrome clinic, I view this illness very differently, I use antipsychotic medications differently, I educate families differently, and I train residents and medical students differently. I think the overarching principle is that the prodrome can be diagnosed, and it is a malignant process that should not be taken, or treated, lightly. (Veteran)

Similarly, residents encountering the psychotic patient in an emergent crisis learn to reframe their understanding of the patient experience:

> I don't know if that helps in terms of self-definition as a psychiatrist, but certainly it's come up a few times; even just calling around to get somebody into a shelter or whatnot. Well, you know, there are all these rules and regulations, and you realize that it's not an easy thing to negotiate and it gives you a lot more empathy for people who have to do this themselves. (Resident)

The veterans and residents that work with patients in the early stages of psychosis learn to redefine their comfort levels with topics related to early intervention. One of the lessons that the veteran clinicians appear to have learned from their work with the early stage psychosis patient was to redefine their comfort with the definition of a good outcome:

> We often say that a patient failed a trial of a treatment or the patient is non-compliant with treatment, the patient is a bad historian. We use language to deflect failure in treatment away from us. And the

prodrome clinic made me face the fact that actually I couldn't help patients in the way I thought I was going to. I now understand that it is sometimes about walking alongside a patient and their families as they learn to include this illness in their lives, rather than trying to focus on whether a hallucination or a delusion has 100% diminished. (Veteran)

Resident clinicians who were in this same situation learned to develop a "comfort zone" in terms of conceptualizing the patient with schizophrenia:

To be able to go and assess a patient who is schizophrenic and not be scared, to dispel illusions that you have about mental illness. It's all about that comfort zone. (Resident)

In the above excerpt, the resident is specifically referring to the need to "dispel illusions" for medical students that work in the psychiatric emergency services. The role of the resident in the relationship with the medical student is primarily a teacher–student relationship and so ensuring that the medical student has an appropriate conceptualization of schizophrenia is important. This is particularly crucial in light of the depictions, and misuses of, the concept of schizophrenia in the general media, which, prior to medical school, might be the primary source for some medical students of information about psychotic disorders.

We Learn about the Importance of Support from Family and Friends

The academic literature describing the family and caregiver experience with the mental health systems suggests that caregivers feel "undervalued" by early intervention teams (Sin, Moore, and Wellman, 2005). The perception of families and caregivers that is described in the literature is contrasted by the depictions of the importance of family and caregiver support described by both early interventionists and residents:

If it wasn't for families, I really think many of my patients would be homeless. It is because of the families that these patients come to the first appointment, come for follow-ups, take medication, and have a roof over their heads during times when they have no money to afford rent anywhere else. Families are just as important as all other aspects of treatment. (Veteran)

Similarly, this resident comments on learning the impact that the presence, and absence, of family support has had on a patient in the emergency room:

You learn about how different people respond to different supports, because you get one patient coming with family members saying they are there for the patient, even while they are crying; then, you see others whose family boots them to be all alone in the ER while they are acutely psychotic, and this person is very sick with no support. So, you see this variety of support, and how people deal with it. (Resident)

Both the residents and the early interventionists describe learning about the importance of being an educator to patients and families. The residents learned this ability through the impact of the acuity of the emergency room presentation:

Things are so much more acute in the emergency room. Patients are so much more worried and frazzled and it makes us more sensitive to the realization that these families are going through a whole lot. Half the time, they don't even know what psychosis is, so you really do have to take the time to explain it to them and be sensitive to that fact. (Resident)

The veterans learned about the importance of patient education not through the acute patient encounter, as the residents did, but, rather, over their long-term relationship with the patient:

So much of the work with patients and families is explaining over and over and over again... Because in early psychosis, the illness teaches the patients. If I stop my meds, I get sick, if I take my meds, I get better. (Veteran)

We Learn How to Deal with Emotional Challenges

The concept of clinician "burnout" is increasingly being recognized in all fields of health care, and the topic is finding coverage on formal training curricula (Maier, 2006). The clinicians in this sample also provided examples of hidden curriculum lessons related to the emotional challenges of practice. What was noticeable about the veteran group were the comments they made in terms of feelings of defeat and loss related to their work with the very early stages of psychosis:

Many of the prodrome patients don't get better. I assess them, I get a sense of their disability, I think I can do something for it, and then six months later, they are still disabled, and I have done nothing. I thought that by intervening in the very early stages, I could do more for these

*patients. Instead, I am watching young, relatively healthy people decline
in front of my eyes. I feel really ineffective. (Veteran)*

The clinician goes on to say:

*I was not prepared for the personal costs, the psychological costs of feel-
ing so defeated in the prodrome clinic. I think I now realize that my
original thought, that this was a prevention clinic, was inaccurate, and
that set me up for failure. I think there could be clinician burnout in
a clinic like this, unless the reality of what it is that we are doing for
patients is clarified. (Veteran)*

The comparison scenario for the residents in the emergency room is
described in the following quotation and is an example in which the resident, similar to the veteran clinician, learns about the importance of managing the difficulties in practice:

*I remember a night, it was one of my first nights, I think, as a second
year and there was this patient with her mom, and they were [threat-
ening] to sue me. She had been in before and she was convinced her
daughter was schizophrenic and needed medications and so on ... I
went home a bit traumatized afterwards ... I think, those nights when
you're kind of just left to yourself when you're having all these difficult
cases and you just go home afterwards and there's really no feed back
about that night. [We need] somebody who is going to say, "OK, that
was obviously schizophrenia; let's do this. (Resident)*

This example also highlights the potential for danger that can be found
in the emergency room when a patient is extremely ill. Given that up to 40
percent of Canadian psychiatry residents in one study reported a physical
assault during training, it can be assumed that assault by a patient is a real
and important clinical challenge that must be managed by the residents
(Chaimowitz and Moscovitch, 1991). While it is generally understood, and
supported by evidence, that there is only a small and complex correlation
between psychosis and violence, the resident working in the emergency
room may encounter the early stage psychosis patient when the illness is
still in an emergent stage, placing the resident in a position where he or she
needs to co-ordinate rapid care (Foley et al., 2007):

*And the patients can be difficult. You may have aggressive patients and
agitated patients, with multiple social issues ... and you have to have*

security there and the nursing staff's all up at arms and can't handle it and, yeah... some of the patients are really difficult. It is mentally and emotionally taxing. It is a different kind of taxing, but the responsibility is quite high. (Resident)

We Learn to Be Honest

James Drane (1995) has written about truth telling by doctors. In his article "Honesty in Medicine: Should Doctors Tell the Truth," Drane (n.d.) comments that "it may be an exaggeration to say that honesty is neither taught in medical school, nor valued in medical culture, but it is not too much of an exaggeration." While the academic literature guides physicians on how to discuss topics such as errors (Hebert, Levin, and Robertson, 2001) and end-stage illness diagnoses with patients (Sloan, 2002), clinicians are rarely taught about how to reveal a serious psychiatric diagnosis to a patient, and it is not included on the list of learning objectives for Canadian psychiatry residency training (RCPSC, 2007a). A patient in Schneider and McDonald's (2008) study commented: "Tell us what is wrong with us. If someone has a heart attack or cancer, you tell them what is wrong with them. But with mental illness, you won't tell us."

Working with the patient in the early stages of psychosis teaches clinicians how to be honest in different ways, depending upon the setting. Residents working in the emergency room must, at times, make the decision to certify a psychotic patient, which is described in the following quotation. This decision requires the resident to inform the patient and family that the patient is not free to leave the hospital and requires an honest and difficult discussion with the clinician:

We anticipate going in for this pretty intensive experience where not only does the patient have to be capable of tolerating what we're asking but we also have to be able to have the resiliency and the fortitude, at three o'clock in the morning, to tactfully and sensitively ask them incredibly personal questions and then, on top of it, occasionally have to make decisions that the patient is not going to like, like removing their rights and admitting them to hospital. It's an incredibly intense, difficult thing. It is really hard and it takes a lot of energy and a lot of focus and it's draining. (Resident)

Veteran clinicians have learned a similar lesson about the need for honesty when facing the decision to explain the diagnosis to an at-risk first episode psychosis patient:

I was thinking about a patient this morning with whom we were not clear about the diagnosis, and we were blaming ourselves and apologizing for not knowing the diagnosis. But in this clinic, it is not always possible to be clear about the diagnosis, and so we monitor mental status, and watch and see. It is such a challenge to monitor a condition that is not described in the main body of the DSM-IV. Frankly, you hope there is not even going to be a diagnosis of schizophrenia, don't you? (Veteran)

Discussion

On the surface, this chapter provides the reader with the opportunity to share reflections on the time spent with, and lessons learned from, our patients. In doing so, we can share the lessons that we have learned, often without always realizing it, from our patients. This chapter began by posing the question: "what can we learn about a person with early stage psychosis if we see the experience from the perspective of the clinicians that care for these patients?" The "lessons learned" by the veterans and residents in this chapter have been taught by the people who have experienced the early stage psychosis first-hand. They are telling us that the person with the very early stages of psychosis:

- faces challenges when dealing with "the system";
- must deal with uncertainty;
- needs more than just a prescription;
- needs us to have an advanced appreciation of his or her experience;
- needs support from family and friends;
- needs us to manage our reaction to this illness; and
- needs our honesty.

This list does not reveal new information, and it concurs with several messages that patients and families have explained, in their own words, to other researchers. Schneider and McDonald (2008) have recently produced what has been described as a poster book, documenting qualitative findings from a participatory action project that was designed to investigate communication between people with schizophrenia and their medical professionals. Participants in this project described, among other themes, challenges with "the system," a need for both biological and non-biological management of their condition, the importance of family, and the need for honesty and clarity from health care providers. The same thoughts are also echoed by the veteran and resident clinicians in this chapter.

It is reassuring that the veteran and novice clinicians who shared their stories in this chapter appear to have an appreciation for the needs and experiences of those who encounter psychosis first-hand. At a deeper level, however, there may be a more complex and interesting phenomena occurring. Why is it that both the resident and veteran clinicians appear to be learning the same lessons from their work with early stage psychosis patients? Should the veterans not already possess the knowledge, skills, and attitudes that the resident clinicians are only beginning to develop? Why does the early stage psychosis patient have a similar and seemingly important impact on clinicians at either end of the spectrum of practice?

One theory to explain the impact of the early stage psychosis patient on the veteran team might be that these clinicians have purposefully defined their area of practice, have an affinity for this patient population, and are more open to hidden curriculum lessons from these encounters. While such an explanation is possible, it does not explain the sense of surprise that the veterans communicated with respect to the lessons they were learning from their patients. Why did their experience in early psychosis intervention not prepare them for the lessons they were learning from the prodrome patients? In other words, why did they not know this information already?

One explanation for the reaction of the resident group might be that the psychotic patient in the emergency room is especially frequent, and therefore, memorable. However, what was interesting about the resident group is that their encounter with the early stage psychosis patient is not necessarily that common. A review of the most common diagnoses listed for patients seen in the Calgary Psychiatric Emergency Services shows that psychosis and schizophrenia appear around the middle of the top ten most common diagnoses. It cannot be argued, therefore, that it is due to the large number of early stage psychosis patients in the emergency room that the residents' experiences with them are particularly impactful or memorable. Nor can it be argued that the presentation of the early stage psychosis patient to the emergency room is so highly unusual that these patients are, by virtue of their rarity, memorable.

So, how might the similarities between the lessons learned by the veterans and residents be explained? One possibility might have to do with the illness and not with the clinicians. In this case, the veterans were not really veterans because they were talking about their experiences establishing a prodrome clinic, which was philosophically, diagnostically, and therapeutically a new way of looking at early intervention. The veterans, despite their experience in standard early psychosis intervention, were forced to learn new knowledge and skills in the management of an unfamiliar patient population. Since residents are physicians-in-training, their encounters with early stage patients serve to develop and continually evolve their knowledge and skills. The veterans and the residents in this case were equalized, such that both groups experienced the relationship with the early stage patients similarly, leading to nearly identical themes. The commonality between the two clinician groups included the need to understand how to be helpful to a patient population with an illness that was not entirely familiar to the clinicians (unfamiliar to the residents because they were still in training and unfamiliar to the veterans because of the emerging aspect of the field). These clinicians shared with their patients similar struggles with a new phenomenon (early stage psychosis) that required adaptation, understanding, and coping. Both the clinicians and the patients must learn to understand and manage the early stages of psychosis, albeit in different ways and for different reasons. With early stage psychosis as the common denominator, the resident and the veterans were trying to understand their role as early intervenors, while the patients were starting to learn what it meant to be a "patient" in a "system." The hidden curriculum in this case might have been the fact that the clinicians identified with the patients' struggle to cope with the early stages of psychosis because the clinicians, too, were adapting to the evolving conditions. Perhaps this mutual struggle is the reason that the patient with early stage psychosis was so impactful (or "memorable," as described by one of the residents) for these clinicians.

The resident and veteran clinicians in this chapter have been talking about what it has been like for them to learn how to help people with schizophrenia. A person presenting for the first time who is in need of treatment for psychosis is starting to learn, for better and for worse, what it means to be a "patient." At the same time, the evolving clinician, often without knowing it, is learning, or being reminded, what it means to be the "doctor," the "case manager," or the "family worker." This resident reflects on the evolution of her role as a care provider in the emergency room:

> It's not only an interesting area but it's rewarding, as well, if you enjoy working with these situations. That's something I've really learned, is that blossoming of how much I enjoy the experience, actually, of these people and getting into people's lives and seeing if you can help them in some way. (Resident)

The early parallels that can be observed between the first episode patient and the resident in their emergency room treatment relationship are simply described by this resident:

I think the psych emerg has the potential to be an incredible place for learning because that's where you see the acuity, right? You see people when they're psychotic...prior to receiving any kind of treatment. So, I think, it is an ideal place to learn. (Resident)

And, finally, this veteran echoes the residents' understanding of the potential lessons that can be learned from working alongside people with early stage psychosis:

It has been very interesting to be one of only a handful of people in the city working with ultra-high-risk groups. The others who have never worked with this population hold many beliefs and assumptions that I remember holding myself two years ago, before we started this clinic. The only way they will start to think differently about how to diagnose or manage the ultra-high-risk person, though, is to try to do it for themselves. The only way they will really understand what this stage of the illness is like is to work with these patients directly. (Veteran)

The valuable lesson to take away from this chapter is that the patient experience is the constant teacher and the clinician must be a lifelong student. No matter how many years of experience the veteran interventionist develops, these data suggest that, in the case of early psychosis, the lessons learned by the novice can be the same as those learned by the early interventionist. This realization is crucial for all early interventionists to remember because of the increasing expectations from both public and international organizations, which are looking to determine measurable outcomes from early intervention teams. The World Health Organization (WHO) and the International Early Psychosis Association (IEPA) (2001) released a joint declaration in 2001 that included a five-year program of action with measurable outcomes by which consumers and teams might gauge the successful and comprehensive implementation of an early intervention program. Included in the recommendations is the acknowledgment that there is a need to develop human resources, both at the level of primary and specialist care. According to the WHO and the IEPA, a "comprehensive program" would include practitioner training that would lead to:

- all primary care sites being equipped to deal effectively with early psychosis;
- continued professional development being supported for all specialist staff working with young people with psychosis;

- the recognition, care, and treatment of young people with psychosis as a routine part of the training curricula for all primary care and social care practitioners; and
- the development of specific early intervention training programs that are resourced and evaluated.

These recommendations mean that consumers and funders of early intervention programs will be asking about how the clinicians in these programs are learning to provide services and care. The WHO and the IEPA have outlined a strategic recommendation that can be followed, depending upon the availability of resources in a community:

> *If resources are low,* then primary care health practitioners must recognise, through awareness training, that young people with psychosis have their own legitimate mental health concerns and needs. There also needs to be awareness training of psychiatrists and nurses about early psychosis care and treatment. *If resource levels are medium,* then specialist mental health practitioners should receive specific training about the recognition, care and treatment of young people with early psychosis. *If resources are high,* then specialist mental health practitioners should develop advanced skills and knowledge about early detection, care and treatment of psychotic disorders in young people. Recognition, care and treatment of young people with psychosis and their families should form a routine part of the training curricula of all primary (generalist) health and social care practitioners. (Ibid., pp. 4-6; emphasis added)

However, the WHO and the IEPA do not advise early interventionists on how to obtain the specific training or advanced skills mentioned in the declaration. It will be relatively simple for early interventionists to create and fulfill stated training objectives. Nonetheless, the findings in this chapter suggest that clinicians that rely solely on stated curricula will neglect important topics because the patient voice (which teaches the hidden curriculum lessons) will not be heard. Primary and specialist care teams interested in developing a full complement of skills to fully serve the person with early stage psychosis might best learn from a combination of a formal curriculum along with regular opportunities for self and group reflection. Many teams may already be familiar with case conferences or team rounds, but, as these meetings tend to degenerate into a discussion of a list of problems for the purpose of diagnosis or treatment decisions, there is a sterilization of the clinician experience in a way in which the patient voice is lost. With the development of a global, online community, reflective discussions may develop through chats and wiki discussions with interventionists around the world or across the city. It will be important to include all members of these teams, at all levels of training, and from all disciplines as well. However, perhaps the best, and the first, place to start hearing the voices of your patients is to answer the question that one of my preceptors from residency would ask any of us after a clinic or a night on call: "Tell me three things you learned from your patients today?"

Acknowledgements

Thank you to Barb Jones and Dora Richardson from the Calgary PRIME clinic for sharing your thoughts about your work with the ultra-high-risk population. Thank you to the University of Calgary Department of Psychiatry residents for sharing your thoughts about your work with patients in the emergency room. Thank you to the Royal College of Physicians and Surgeons of Canada for funding the study of the resident experience in the emergency department.

References

American Psychiatric Association. (2000). *Diagnostic and statistical manual of mental disorders* (4th edition).

Borkan, J.M. (1999). Crystallization-immersion. In B. Crabtree and W. Miller (Eds.), *Doing Qualitative Research* (2nd ed.). London: Sage Publications.

Borkan, J., Reis, S., Steinmetz, D., and Medalie, J. (1999). *Patients and doctors: Life changing stories from primary care.* Madison, WI: University of Wisconsin Press.

Brasch, J.S., and Ferencz, J.C. (1999). Training issues in emergency psychiatry. *Psychiatric Clinics of North America, 22*(4), 941-54.

Brodkey, A., Van Zant. K., and Sieries, F. (1997). Educational objectives for a junior psychiatry clerkship. *Academic Psychiatry, 21,* 179-204.

Canadian Association of Emergency Physicians (CAEP). (2007). *CAEP Statement: Emergency department overcrowding.* Online: http://www.caep.ca.

Chaimowitz, G.A., and Moscovitch, A. (1991). Patient assaults on psychiatric residents: The Canadian experience. *Canadian Journal of Psychiatry, 36,* 107-11.

Department of Psychiatry, University of Calgary. (N.d.). *Learning Objectives for Early Psychosis Fellowship.* Online: http://www.ucalgary.ca.

Dowling, A., and Engel, G. (2005). *American Journal of Psychiatry, 162*(11), 1913-99.

Drane, J.F. (1995). *Becoming a good doctor: The place of virtue and character in medical ethics* (2nd edition). Kansas City, MO: Sheed and Ward.

Drane, J.F. (n.d.). Honesty in medicine: Should doctors tell the truth? Online: http://www.uchile.cl/bioetica/doc/honesty.htm.

Foley, Sr., Browne, S., Clarke, M., Kinsella, A., Larkin, C., and O'Callaghan, E. (2007). Is violence at presentation by patients with first-episode psychosis associated with duration of untreated psychosis? *Social Psychiatry Psychiatric Epidemiology, 42*(8), 606-10.

Hebert, P., Levin, A., and Robertson, G. (2001). Bioethics for clinicians: Disclosure of medical error. *Canadian Medical Association Journal, 164*(4), 509-13.

Holmqvist, R. (1998). The influence of patient diagnosis and self-image on clinicians' feelings. *Journal of Nervous Mental Disease, 186*(8), 455-61.

Killackey, E., Yung, A., and McGorry, P. (2007). Early psychosis: Where we've been, where we still have to go. *Journal of Epidemiology and Psychiatric Sciences, 16*(2), 102-8.

Lam, V. (2006). *Bloodletting and other miraculous cures.* Mississauga, ON: Random House.

Lempp, H., and Seale, C. (2004). The hidden curriculum in undergraduate medical education: Qualitative study of medical student's perception of teaching. *British Medical Journal, 329,* 770-73.

Maier, D.B. (2006). Finding your groove in a group: Physician support groups. *Alberta Doctor's Digest.* Online: http://www.albertadoctors.org/bcm/ama/amawebsite.nsf/AllDoc/C9533AA3EB92B7D887257103005C7C98/$File/Finding_your_groove_janfeb_06.pdf.

Pekkanen, J. (1988). *Doctors talk about themselves.* New York: Delacourte Press.

Reame, J. (2002). From lunatic to patient to person: Nomenclature in psychiatric history and the influence of patients' activism in North America. *International Journal of Law and Psychiatry, 25,* 405-26.

Royal College of Physians and Surgeons of Canada (RCPSC). (2007a). *Specialty training requirements in psychiatry.* Online: http://www.rcpsc.medical.org.

RCPSC. (2007b). *Specific standards of accreditation for residency programs in psychiatry.* Online: http://www.rcpsc.medical.org.

Schneider, B., and McDonald, C. (2008). *Schizophrenia: Hearing [our] voices, dilemmas of care and control.* Calgary, AB: University of Calgary.

Sin, J., Moore, N., and Wellman, N. (2005). Developing services for the carers of young adults with early onset psychosis: Listening to their experiences and needs. *Journal of Psychiatric and Mental Health Nursing, 12*(5), 589-97.

Sloan, R. (2002). Cancer isn't the only malignant disease. *British Medical Journal, 324*(7344), 1035.

World Health Organization and International Early Psychosis Association. (2001). *Early Psychosis Declaration: An international consensus statement about early intervention and recovery for young people with psychosis.* Online: http://www.iris-initiative.org.uk/silo/files/early-psychosis-declaration.pdf.

6

Promoting Constructive Change in the Service System: A Qualitative Study of Change in Staff Attitudes with the Implementation of Early Intervention in Psychosis

Alan Rosen, Joanne Gorrell, Alison Cornish, Vivienne Miller, Chris Tennant, Louise Nash, and Dianne McKay

Introduction

The past decade has seen a significant shift in mental health services towards an early intervention approach to the treatment of first episode psychosis (FEP). The introduction of such a new approach to service provision requires that individual clinicians change their practices in order for the new approach to be available to all who may benefit. Obstacles to change can include a lack of information and skill as well as attitudinal barriers, particularly if the new approach represents a significant change from established practices. How the front-line user feels about and perceives change will largely determine whether change occurs and how successful the change process may be (Hall and Hord, 1987).

Innovation diffusion theory attempts to identify the factors that facilitate the adoption of new practices (Rogers, 1983). Specific features of a proposed innovation are predicted to be associated with positive attitudes in those who will be involved in the change. These features include: (1) relative advantage: the degree to which an innovation is perceived to be better than the current practice; (2) compatibility: the degree to which an innovation is perceived to be consistent with the existing values of the potential adopters; (3) complexity: the degree to which an innovation is perceived to be relatively difficult to understand and use; (4) trialability; and (5) observability (ibid.). Factor analyses of the perceptions of teachers and farmers about new ideas found the strongest support for the dimensions of relative advantage, compatibility, and complexity (ibid.). Therefore, the degree to which the early intervention approach is simple, consistent with current beliefs and practice, and more effective should be associated with its adoption by clinicians.

A Clinician's Dilemma: Change versus Conservation

Change in clinical service systems is required in response to emerging evidence of better practice, including interventions and delivery systems with better outcomes. However, change should also spring to life as part of a perpetual tango with conservation. We should conserve ways of working that are worth keeping because they are tried, tested, and remain true. Clinicians are constantly confronted with the dilemma of what to change and what to keep, and they sometimes find it hard to keep their balance when they are caught up in the dance between the two options.

While the delivery of health care is growing more complex, no other clinical specialty has encountered change on such a scale as Western mental health service systems (Callaly and Arya, 2005). Drivers for such change include shifts from institutional to community care, pressure for better integration of services, new technologies, the rise of the consumer, family and recovery movements, human rights awareness, and the public health movement, which is promoting proactive early detection, engagement, assessment, and intervention.

Clinicians want to change things for the better for their clientele, but they are frequently skeptical about an endless stream of initiatives imposed from above. They see no clear purpose in following incoherent or conflicting directions for change and sometimes have serious concerns about the way in which changes are implemented (Callaly and Arya, 2005; Golop, Whitby, Buchanan, and Kentley, 2004). Effective change requires a "learning organization," with effective leadership and an organizational culture that promotes creativity, risk taking, reflection, and new learning (Senge, 1990). As such, staff at every level should make sense of the changed way of working and claim some personal ownership of it.

Clinicians' Attitudes to Practice Innovation

The influences on clinicians to change their clinical practices were studied by mapping doctors' attitudes in semi-structured interviews to the implementation of new clinical practice guidelines (Hader et al., 2007). Using an innovation theory framework, doctors identified that any decisions to change their practices were not simple. Such decisions were made in response to diverse and complex factors and influences, including the finding that their perceived need to change depends on the evidence of better outcomes without more risk and also on the basis of opinion leader support and consistency with current trends; how well the awareness of need for change is communicated clearly or taught to the clinician; and whether it is acceptable to, and supported by, both patients and families. Families, service users, and professional networks will support such change strongly if they have personally or collectively observed improved patient outcomes without increased risk. Practice innovation—for example, in primary care—can be shown to be associated with better team climates, which predict higher job satisfaction, and is correlated with separate but connected sub-cultures between clinical and administrative staff (Proudfoot et al., 2007).

Clinicians' Attitudes to Mental Health Innovations

Approval by fellow health workers, including doctors and service users, of trials using nurses to prescribe medications in psychiatry appear to be dependent on fellow professionals having experienced this innovation at close quarters and to be evidence-based, person-centred, clinically focused, and additionally focused on physical health (Jones, Bennett, Lucas, Miller, and Gray, 2007). Successful change in the utilization of nurses who were institutionally based rather than those who were based in mobile community mental health practices was related to the value of exercising increased professional autonomy taking more moral responsibility for service users, while not intruding on service-user autonomy (Magnussen, Hogberg, Lutzen, and Severinsson, 2004). However, training in adopting a health outcomes approach, and in outcome measurement techniques, improved the potential for health gains in the clientele of community mental health professionals (Crocker and Rissel, 1998).

Clinicians' Attitudes to Consumer Initiatives

With respect to the evaluation of clinicians' attitudes to the implementation of psychiatric advance directives ("living wills"), there were significant differences between disciplines (Van Dorn et al., 2006). Psychiatrists perceived more obstacles than other professions and were much more likely to perceive more clinical barriers, while all professionals perceived some operational barriers.

Mental health professionals were found to have favourable attitudes towards consumer participation in management, care, and treatment on several different types of psychiatric inpatient units, though they were less supportive of such participation when it impinged on their spheres of professional responsibility (McCann, Laird, Clark, and Lui, 2006). Support from postgraduate psychiatric nursing students for the involvement of a consumer academic in their education was found to increase after they were exposed to the consumer academic (Happell, Marti, and Pinikahana, 2003).

Clinicians' Attitudes to Evidence-Based Practice (EBP)

Gregory Aarons (2004) derived four dimensions of attitudes towards the adoption of EBP in public mental health workers: its intuitive appeal, the likelihood of implementation being required, its openness to new practices, and the perceived divergence of usual practice from EBP. Provider attitudes were found to vary by educational level, level of experience, and organizational context, with lower levels of bureaucracy being more conducive to the adoption of EBPs.

Effect of Clinicians' Training on Attitudes

Following a six-hour workshop for general practitioners (GPs) on mental health assessment, intervention, and clinical management planning, there was an increased use by GPs of psycho-education, cognitive behaviour therapy, and expert clinical advice (Hodgins, Judd, Davis, and Faley, 2007).

Clinicians' Attitudes to Early Intervention in Psychosis Innovations

A sample of GPs in East Dublin were highly receptive to the implementation of an early intervention in psychosis service on the basis that this service model promised to reduce the challenges of managing psychosis in primary care, including the practical difficulties of accessing psychiatric assessment and of overcoming stigma. The GPs viewed communication between primary and specialist care as being essential to the success of this innovation (Gavin et al., 2008). The attitudes of consultant psychiatrists were mixed regarding the proposed implementation of specialist teams, including early intervention in the psychosis teams. Half of them indicated that such teams would provide a welcome change of role for psychiatrists, reduce admissions, and increase patient satisfaction, while the other half were concerned that the resources were insufficient and that these services would be developed at the expense of existing teams (Harrison, McKay, and Bannon, 2004).

A pilot study of a partnership approach used to help existing primary and secondary mental health staff adapt to working with teams delivering an early intervention in psychosis service demonstrated that the surrounding staff showed an improvement in their knowledge, attitudes, and professional practices that was compatible with their confidence in this innovation (Paxton et al., 2003).

As in other mental health services, early intervention services and practitioners' ambivalence towards the families of their patients may contribute to the limited development of specific interventions for these families (Askey, Gamble, and Gray, 2007). Clinicians' attitudes to the delivery of early intervention in psychosis may be vastly improved by specific training in relevant psychosocial (including family) intervention skills (Brabban and Kelly, 2008; Fadden and Palmer, 2008). Particular needs for training and support of more isolated early intervention practitioners in rural settings has also been addressed (Kelly, O'Meara, Howard, and Smith 2007).

Triangulation and Stages of Concern: A Qualitative and Quantitative Study of a Regional Early Intervention in Psychosis Initiative

Setting: Northern Sydney Health Area Mental Health Services
Northern Sydney Health (NSH) Area Mental Health Service, which deals with a population of 750,000, is comprised of four sectors, each including an acute inpatient unit, a consultation liaison service, and an integrated twenty-four hour community mental health service providing acute and long-term care, child and adolescent services, aged care services, rehabilitation, and residential services. Recent years have witnessed a reorientation of the NSH's Mental Health Services towards a systematic early intervention approach to psychosis, without any additional funding. Over this period, all staff in the local sector mental health services were offered orientation and training programs. Services were restructured to develop three early intervention teams and a dedicated respite residential facility, and national guidelines were operationalized to promote best practice for early psychosis services. Following this restructuring, a project officer was employed to liaise with teams and utilize a consultative approach to develop manuals of local clinical guidelines with concomitant staff training for every component of the new service. Since 2005, this area's mental health service has been merged with its neighbouring area—the Central Coast—and now has four local early intervention in psychosis teams. In 2007, the Central Coast became the first pilot program in the state for an integrated "one-stop-shop" youth health centre approach to early intervention. In 2011, due to federally mandated changes in health delivery organizations, these services reverted yet again into the separate Northern Sydney and Central Coast Local Health Districts.

Research Program
The introduction of early intervention services for young people with psychosis in the NSH's Mental Health Services has been evaluated by the research arm of the Early Psychosis Prevention and Intervention Network

for Young People (EPPINY). A multiple triangulated research approach was adopted to increase confidence in the quality of findings from a combination of the quasi-experimental assessment of client outcomes (Nash et al., 2004) and empirical auditing (Gorrell et al., 2004a; McKay et al., 2006) and a qualitative study of staff perceptions and attitudes, which were expected to implement early intervention in psychosis protocols (Gorrell et al., 2002; Rosen et al., 2007). A parallel study examined subjective perceptions of pathways and obstacles to care experienced by individuals and families and their clinical implications (Gorrell et al., 2004b; Moss and Gorrell, 2006).

Objectives

Our objectives were twofold: (1) to determine the perceptions, attitudes, and concerns of health professionals regarding the introduction of an early intervention approach to the treatment of psychosis using both qualitative and quantitative inquiry and (2) to measure changes in attitudes and concerns as an indication of the success of a service development program, in parallel and in triangulation with empirical studies of the fidelity and effectiveness of the implementation of an early intervention in psychosis program using both qualitative and quantitative inquiry.

Method

Triangulation of method was employed as a mode of inquiry intrinsic to qualitative research (Huberman and Miles, 1994, p. 438; Miles and Huberman, 1984) and was originally classified into four basic types based on the data source, investigator, theory, and method (Denzin, 1978). Triangulated analysis of data related to similar constructs generated by qualitative and quantitative methods that provide both convergent validity and a broader understanding of the subject matter that contributes to both verification and completeness (Breitmayer, Ayres, and Knafi, 1993). Multiple triangulation is defined as the combination of any two or more types of triangulation in one study, which occurred in the study in this chapter (Kimchi, Polivka, and Stevensen, 1991).

Questionnaire Development

The Perceptions of Early Psychosis Intervention (PEPI) questionnaire was developed and distributed to all clinicians in NSH's Mental Health Services at three time points at eighteen-month intervals (see Appendix 1). The PEPI questionnaire was designed to collect both quantitative (Part A) and qualitative (Part B) data.

1. The initial item pool was generated following consultation with service providers and guided by the literature regarding the diffusion of innovations, mental health service change, and the benefits of early intervention.
2. Experts rated items for relevance and clarity, with some items being discarded and additional items being added.
3. A pilot questionnaire, comprising forty-one self-statements was administered to eighty clinicians from hospital and community mental health services.
4. Exploratory factor analyses and reliability analyses were conducted for each theoretically derived factor to eliminate items. Items that were unclear or were not discriminating were removed. Concurrent validity was examined by contrasting total scores of two groups of respondents understood to have different attitudes towards early intervention (participants in early psychosis workshops versus untrained inpatient staff). Mean scores were, as expected, greatest for the respondents who had recently participated in an early psychosis training workshop (n = 21, mean = 115, standard deviation = 8.75) and lowest for those working in an inpatient unit (n = 7, mean = 102, standard deviation = 6.8).

Part A of the PEPI questionnaire consists of ratings from twenty-six self-statements on a five-point Likert scales contributing to four scales: compatibility of early psychosis intervention (EPI) with (1) the respondents' general beliefs, (2) perceived advantages and disadvantages of the intervention, (3) readiness to provide early intervention, and (4) current adoption of early intervention principles. These scales were based on and modified from Everett Rogers' (1983) theoretically and empirically derived dimensions. The standardized item alpha for the remaining four scales were .66, .89, .82, and .88 respectively.

Part B outlines clinicians' concerns, which were elicited by their responses to an open-ended concerns statement adapted from Gene Hall and Shirley Hord (1987): "When you think about the implementation of special intervention strategies for early psychosis in your services what are your concerns?" Participants provided a written response in the space provided on the questionnaire. Clinicians' written responses were analyzed according to the "stages of concern" (SoC) methodology. The SoC method encodes individual statements of respondents' concerns about an innovation according to four developmental stages—informational, self, task, and impact related, with a preceding stage of little or unrelated concerns. These categories were adapted from Hall and Hord (1987), following the guidelines of Beulah Newlove and Hall (1998) (see Table 1). Each concern was coded for its stage of development and then subjected to content analysis.

TABLE 1: STAGES OF CONCERN

	STAGE	DESCRIPTION
1	Unrelated	Little concern about, and involvement with, the new innovation
2	Information	General awareness and interest in learning more about the innovation
3	Self	Uncertain about the demands of the new approach and the best use of information and resources
4	Task	Focused on the processes and tasks of using the new approach and the best use of information and resources
5	Impact	Focused on how the new approach is affecting clients and how service provision can be improved

Source: Adapted from Hall and Hord (1987).

Ethical Considerations

Ethics approval for the study was obtained from all relevant area ethics committees. While verbal consent was sought, respondents were advised that completion of the questionnaire would constitute formal consent for participation in the research project.

Scoring and Data Analysis

- PEPI Part A on attitudes and beliefs about the introduction of EPI using the PEPI questionnaire: Likert scale items were scored from one (strongly disagree) to five (strongly agree), with the exception of two items, which were reverse scored. Averaged item response scores for each scale score were calculated for the overall sample. These responses provide an indication of the extent to which clinicians held beliefs likely to lead to their adoption of early psychosis intervention.
- PEPI Part B on the stages of concern: Each concern was coded according to the five developmental stages defined by Hall et al. (1979) and Hall and Hord (1987) as unrelated, information, self, task, or impact (see Table 1), following the guidelines set out by Newlove and Hall (1998). The percentages of concerns in each developmental stage were calculated for each of the three time points. Subcategories were then created for each task and impact concern in order to provide more specific information to inform service developments.

Results

Sample

Responses were completed by 143, 178, and 102 staff at Time 1, Time 2, and Time 3. Response rates were 35 percent, 46 percent, and 25 percent respectively. A proportion of the sample is comprised of repeated measures with forty-six clinicians identified as responding at both Time 1 and Time 2 and thirty-six responding at both Time 2 and Time 3. Only thirteen clinicians responded at all three time points. The majority of respondents at each time point were working in community (28 percent), rehabilitation (30 percent), or in-patient (20 percent) settings. The proportion of respondents working in specialized early psychosis teams increased from 2 percent (n = 3) at Time 1 to 11 percent in the Time 3 period as these teams developed.

Attitudes and Beliefs about the Introduction of Early Psychosis Intervention

Descriptive Statistics for Total Sample

On average, respondents agreed with statements of beliefs that were compatible with an early intervention approach. This finding was consistent across time. At all three time points, respondents from early psychosis teams agreed more strongly than other respondents, and those from in-patient units responded least strongly. The only change over time appears to be in the early psychosis and child and adolescent teams. Early psychosis team respondents rated these statements less favourably at Time 1 and Time 2 than at Time 2. This finding could be due to the very small sample of enthusiastic clinicians at the first time point. Child and adolescent workers also gradually rated these statements less favourably over time.

Overall, a similar pattern was observed for statements about the specific advantages of an early intervention approach with average responses falling consistently across time and service type at "agree." Within this category, early intervention teams rated these statements most favourably and in-patient staff rated them least favourably. Child and adolescent workers rated these statements more favourably at the two later time points than they did initially.

At all three time points, on average, respondents were undecided about their readiness to provide early psychosis intervention. However, perceived readiness varied for clinicians from different service settings. As expected, respondents from early psychosis teams agreed or strongly agreed that they had sufficient training and skills and were currently able to provide early psychosis intervention. In contrast, clinicians working in rehabilitation

FIGURE 1: PEPI RESULTS FOR EACH SCALE AT TIME 1, TIME 2, AND TIME 3

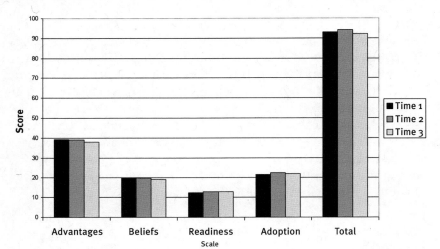

settings, aged-care facilities, and in-patient units were clearly undecided. Respondents from child and adolescent services rated these statements less favourably over time (from agree to undecided to disagree). Item analysis indicates that at Time 3 these clinicians indicated that they did not have sufficient training available to them and were not able to provide early intervention for psychosis.

In contrast to readiness, the average response to statements about the current adoption of early psychosis practices was "agreed." This finding did not change over time. As expected, early psychosis teams rated these items more favourably (agree to strongly agree) than other groups. Item analyses revealed that respondents agreed most strongly that their service provides family support and education (72 percent agreed or strongly agreed). Community awareness training was perceived to be least well adopted (45 percent agreed or strongly agreed that their service provided this training).

Repeated Measures Data
For a sub-sample of forty-six clinicians who completed the questionnaire at both Time 1 and Time 2 data, paired t-test analyses indicated that at the second time point they rated themselves and their colleagues as more able to provide early psychosis interventions (Scale 3: $t = -3.38$, degrees of freedom $= 43$, $p < .005$) and their services more adopting of Early Psychosis Intervention principles (Scale 4: $t = -2.95$, degrees of freedom $= 38$, $p < .01$).

FIGURE 2: CLINICIAN CONCERNS FOR EACH SCALE AT TIME 1, TIME 2, AND TIME 3

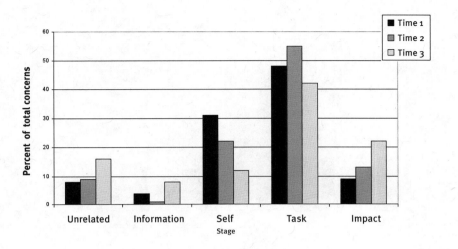

Clinicians' Concerns

Comparison of Developmental Stage of Clinicians' Concerns from Time 1 and Time 2 to Time 3
The number of concerns expressed at each time interval were 193, 239, and 139. Results indicate a progression up the developmental stages of the stages of concern model (see Figure 2). The proportion of concerns that were about self (how will the change affect me?) decreased (from 31 percent, to 22 percent, to 12 percent). Task-related concerns (that is, about the practicalities of getting the job done) increased over time from 48 percent to 55 percent and then reduced to 42 percent. Impact concerns (is it working and how can we do it better?) increased from an initial 9 percent, to 13 percent, and then to 22 percent. Analyses of specific content of concerns were used to guide the change process.

Content Analyses of Concerns
At all three times, more than 40 percent of respondents' concerns were at the task level—that is, clinicians were mostly concerned about the actual process of providing EPI to clients. The content of task concerns was therefore examined, and five subcategories were identified (see Figure 3):

1. Management: these concerns were mostly regarding a perceived lack of support, direction, and implementation. With respect to resources, concerns were about insufficient resources and resource allocation.

FIGURE 3: CONTENT OF TASK CONCERNS

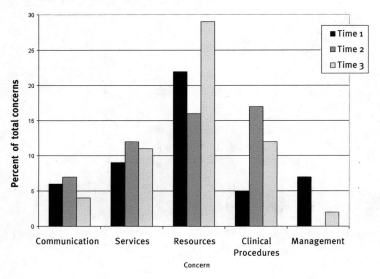

2. Clinical procedures: these concerns were mostly about consistent implementation of specific interventions. With respect to services, these concerns were mostly about gaps in services.
3. Inter-team communication: these concerns primarily dealt with a lack of communication, specifically what happens on the acute unit and after discharge.

From Time 1 to Time 2, concerns about management and resources decreased while concerns about clinical procedures and services increased. At Time 2, the greatest number of concerns were about resources and clinical procedures. At Time 3, there was a further increase in concerns about resources, such as time for administrative responsibilities, funding needed for additional cars and staff, which was accompanied by a decrease in the concerns about clinical procedures (managing substance use, the need for treatment guidelines) and inter-team communication.

Impact concerns increased over time to more than 20 percent of the concerns expressed at Time 3. The content of impact concerns was examined and found to include:

1. What comes next: these concerns deal with what happens to clients after eighteen months of treatment and the fact that the transition to general adult mental health services needs to be improved.

2. Expectations: these concerns relate to the fact that clients and families from early psychosis teams have expectations of a level of treatment that cannot be provided in general adult mental health services.
3. Potential benefits to other client groups: these concerns involve clients outside the strict criteria of the early psychosis teams who may also benefit from early intervention especially when a first episode occurs prior to the age of eighteen (or sixteen if not still in school).
4. Evidence: these concerns consider whether what the individuals are doing is really making a difference to the client's mental health?
5. Alternatives: suggestions of other treatment strategies that may augment early intervention.

Discussion

Studies of the impact of staff reorientation and retraining are still a relative rarity in this field, and it is essential that we understand their implications so that we can improve and sustain such reskilling processes and outcomes. In a real-world implementation action research study, triangulation of method can provide more confidence for a trend in findings by demonstrating that independent measures or methods agree or at least do not contradict it. It can also overcome or circumvent the effect of observational or interactional bias. General practitioners, car mechanics, and detectives are all able to establish and corroborate findings with little elaborate instrumentation. They often use a *"modus operandi"* approach— triangulating different kinds of independent indices. The triangulating researcher self-consciously sets out to collect and double-check findings, using multiple sources and modes of evidence to build the triangulation process into an ongoing mode of inquiry (Huberman and Miles, 1994).

Clinicians' Attitudes

Little published data was found addressing clinicians' attitudes to EPI or on the impact of change strategies on staff attitudes, nor were there any suitable assessment instruments available. The present study utilized both diffusion theory and concerns theory to develop a questionnaire that would both explore staff attitudes and examine and facilitate the process of change (Hall and Hord, 1987; Rogers, 1983). The PEPI questionnaire was developed to determine the attitudes and concerns of clinicians towards the introduction of an EPI approach to the care of FEP.

Initial attitudes that were determined from self-ratings by clinicians indicated that, on average, respondents held beliefs that were consistent with an early intervention approach. Most respondents indicated that they expected early intervention to provide better outcomes for clients and families, although such intervention would not necessarily be more cost-effective or beneficial for staff. Respondents were undecided about their own readiness to provide early psychosis intervention. Responses suggested that barriers to implementation included a lack of knowledge or skills rather than a poor attitude towards the subject. Respondents from Child and Adolescent Services rated these statements less favourably over time, which may reflect less direct involvement with the early psychosis teams and possibly less commitment or capacity to work in this way.

Attitudes and concerns determined at the two subsequent time points, which were both eighteen months apart, provided a measure of change and, therefore, an indication of the success of the service development strategies in promoting the change process. At the first time point, one-third of concerns were about self, indicating that these clinicians were seeking information and considering how the change would affect them. However, 48 percent of concerns were already about getting on with the task and 8 percent were about the impact of the change process, indicating that for these clinicians practices had already begun to change. The concerns-based adoption model provides a means to assess and catalogue staff perceptions. Content analyses identified common concerns. At this time point, the majority of task concerns were about resources, particularly those resources that might be allocated to this innovation at the expense of longer-term clients. Other concerns were about gaps in services, inter-team communication, clinical procedures, and a lack of management support. In addition, a common theme involved a liaison with, and provision of, services in the in-patient unit.

Clinicians' Concerns: Stages of Concern

"Concerns" theory provides the facilitators of a new innovation with ways to assess and catalogue the different perceptions of the staff during the introduction of a new innovation. The concept of "concerns" emerged in the late 1960s from the work of Frances Fuller in the area of teacher training. Fuller identified and described four major clusters of concerns (unrelated, self, task, and impact) that have subsequently been verified, modified, and adapted by other researchers. SoC is a dimension of the concerns-based adoption model (Hall, Wallace, and Dossett, 1973), which was devised for the education sector but can be effectively applied to any sector experiencing change (for example, Hall et al., 1979; Hall and Hord, 1987; Hord, 1987; Hord, Rutherford, Huling-Austin, and Hall, 1987). The SoC method has been applied to a variety of innovations such as exercise (Jordan-Marsh, 1985), computer technology (Lewis and Watson, 1997; McKinnon and Nolan, 1989), education (Gwele, 1996), and diabetes (Lewis, 1996), but, to our knowledge, it has rarely been applied to clinicians' attitudinal adaptation to innovation in a mental health setting. Its first widely known published application was a mental health quality improvement study (Anderson and Forquer, 1982), which exemplified the use of SoC methodology as a candidate tool in applying Australian national mental health standards (Miller, Rosen, Parker, and Hartley, 1991).

The SoC model reflects empirically based developmental stages that individuals are hypothesized to move through as they become increasingly familiar with, and skilled in, applying a new approach. These stages are based on the finding that individuals have concerns during the process of adopting a new approach and that specific types of concerns are more intense at different times in the change process. The stages range from early "self"-type concerns (for example, feeling unsure about the demands of the new approach on me, my time, and my personal resources as a service provider), to "task" concerns, which address the logistics with regard to the use of the innovation, and ultimately to "impact" concerns, which evaluate and increase the effectiveness of the innovation (Hall and Hord, 1987). The model assumes that change is an ongoing process rather than a discrete event and that the identification of concerns can be used to develop appropriate interventions to facilitate the change process. The provision of support activities can, therefore, be designed to address clinicians' concerns and promote the effective and skilled application of the new approach. Thus, in disseminating a new approach, change facilitators must address attitude, knowledge, and skills. A consultative approach to change, including the opportunity for staff to express their values and their concerns, is recommended.

Analysis of clinicians' concerns according to the stages of concern model revealed a progression leading up through the developmental stages of the model from self to the task at hand and its impact. There was a gradual resolution of self-concerns to only 13 percent at Time 3. Task concerns, which were the most common at all three time points, peaked at Time 2 with a reduction in concerns about inter-team communication, services, and clinical procedures at Time 3. Concerns about resources remained high but shifted to concerns about the adequacy of resources rather than resource allocation. Specifically, at Time 3, clinicians wanted funds for additional cars and staff. Impact concerns increased to 22 percent at Time 3. The focus of these concerns was on providing an optimal level of care after clients have received the eighteen months of service provided by specialized early psychosis teams and on demonstrating outcomes.

For those clinicians who responded to the questionnaire on more than one occasion, there was a shift from Time 1 to Time 2 in their perception of themselves as being more able to provide EPI and of their services as being more capable of adopting early psychosis principles. Descriptive data indicate that these shifts also occurred for the overall sample. There was no change in the compatibility of beliefs or in the perceived advantage of early intervention for the overall sample, although agreement with these items remained high.

It is likely that these shifts towards a more favourable attitude to early intervention are the outcome of the use of educational programs and service restructuring, which took place as dissemination strategies during the thirty-six-month period. Evidence of management support for the innovation, particularly service restructuring during Time 1 and the employment of a project officer after Time 2 who was able to provide face-to-face encouragement, are factors that are likely to have contributed to the resolution of personal concerns by Time 3 (Hall and Hord, 1987). Task concerns became more intense at the second time point, which coincided with the time when all three specialized teams were in operation and significant changes in service provision had occurred (Gorrell et al., 2004a). This increase in task concerns when the innovation was first implemented was expected. Some resolution of these task concerns by Time 3 is a likely outcome of further, more targeted training sessions, location visits by the project officer, coaching and consulting, and the development and provision of clinical guidelines.

The resolution of self and task concerns are indications of success in implementing an innovation. The arousal of impact concerns indicates that staff had become concerned about the outcomes and were collaborating to work more effectively. In order to develop conditions that will stimulate impact concerns, it is considered that management support must be developed over at least three to five years (Hall and Hord, 1987). At the time of writing, it is twelve years since the onset of this project. Ongoing management support has been demonstrated by the extension of the inclusion criteria for the early psychosis teams to work with clients for three years rather than eighteen months, a widening of the eligible age group to between sixteen and thirty years of age, and the continuing appointment of an area-wide (now local health district-wide) early intervention co-ordinator to extend the work conducted by the project officer. This position, along with the continuation of regular EPPINY meetings, have provided the vehicle by which further collaborative work can occur. It is this work that is most likely to further arouse progress up the developmental stages to concerns about impact (Hall and Hord, 1987).

Conclusion

To our knowledge, this chapter represents the first study to apply diffusion theory or the Stages of Concern model to the introduction of innovation in early psychosis intervention or even to study clinicians' concerns in parallel with the attitudes of staff. This data has been valuable in enabling the Northern Sydney Health (NSH) Area Mental Health Service Early Psychosis Program to address clinicians' concerns and further facilitate the change process.

The aim of this study was to ascertain the attitudes, views, and concerns regarding EPI of clinicians from all teams comprising an integrated community and hospital mental health service prior to and after the implementation of change strategies. Change strategies included staff training, service restructuring, and the development of local clinical guidelines. Specifically, this study evaluated the effectiveness of our approach to the introduction of innovation in early psychosis treatment as measured at three time points by:

- the beliefs held by staff about the relative advantage, compatibility, complexity, and practicality of the approach; and
- stages of concerns among clinicians about the introduction of an EPI approach.

The PEPI questionnaire appears to be a useful instrument for assessing staff attitudes and concerns. There has been a small shift towards a more favourable attitude towards providing EPI. Paired time tests used to compare ratings of self-statements indicated an increase from Time 1 to Time 2 in health professionals' perceptions of their own ability to provide early psychosis interventions and their services' adoption of early psychosis principles. Overall, respondents generally agreed with statements regarding the general and specific advantages of early psychosis intervention (EPI), were undecided about their own readiness to provide EPI, and some uncertainty remained regarding whether their services had yet to fully adopted EPI.

In terms of the stages of concern methodology, clinicians' concerns moved up the developmental stages from focus on the self, to the task, and then to the impact of the intervention service subsystem. Data have been helpful in enabling NSH to address clinicians' concerns throughout the change process, and the entire initiative has been sustained and is continuing to develop. Furthermore, content analyses of qualitative information from the first and second surveys will assist in the planning of training as well as in the provision of a baseline for subsequent evaluations. It is anticipated that the questionnaire developed for this study will prove useful for adaptation by other services undergoing change.

PERCEPTIONS OF EARLY PSYCHOSIS INTERVENTION

The implementation in our services of strategies for early intervention for psychosis:

	strongly disagree	disagree	undecided	agree	strongly agree
1. Will lead to significantly improved recovery for early psychosis clients	1	2	3	4	5
2. Will significantly reduce disruption to educational and vocational paths of early psychosis clients	1	2	3	4	5
3. Will significantly reduce disruption to social and family relationships	1	2	3	4	5
4. Will significantly improve overall client outcomes	1	2	3	4	5
5. Will lead to a significant reduction in co-morbidity (such as depression, anxiety, and substance use)	1	2	3	4	5
6. Will reduce the long-term economic costs of pychosis to the community	1	2	3	4	5
7. Can improve the course of illness for young people with early psychosis	1	2	3	4	5
8. Will significantly benefit clients with their first episode of psychosis	1	2	3	4	5
9. Will improve staff enthusiasm and satisfaction	1	2	3	4	5
10. Will help to increase clients hopefulness about their future	1	2	3	4	5
11. The early intervention approach to psychosis is a multifaceted, comprehensive approach	1	2	3	4	5
12. The early intervention approach to psychosis offers nothing new to usual knowledge and practice	1	2	3	4	5
13. Sufficient training and information is available for my team to be able to develop the clinical skills for intervention in early psychosis	1	2	3	4	5
14. I currently have the clinical knowledge and skills to provide interventions to young people with early psychosis	1	2	3	4	5
15. I am currently able within my service to conduct intervention for young people with early psychosis	1	2	3	4	5
16. I have received sufficient training to be able to provide interventions to young people with early psychosis	1	2	3	4	5
17. The recent focus on early intervention represents significant progress in the way we assist individuals with psychosis	1	2	3	4	5

	strongly disagree	disagree	undecided	agree	strongly agree
18. Research findings indicate that existing services for young people with early psychosis can be significantly improved	1	2	3	4	5
19. Research findings indicate that existing services for young people with early psychosis can be significantly improved	1	2	3	4	5
20. The effort involved in taking on such initiatives is rarely worthwhile	1	2	3	4	5

In my service, intervention for young people with early psychosis is currently guided by the following principles:

21. "User friendly" service for young people	1	2	3	4	5
22. Community awareness training about the need for early intervention	1	2	3	4	5
23. Low-dose medication	1	2	3	4	5
24. Intensive, assertive case management	1	2	3	4	5
25. Individual therapeutic / psychological management	1	2	3	4	5
26. Family support and education	1	2	3	4	5

PLEASE TAKE A FEW MINUTES TO ANSWER THIS FINAL QUESTION

When you think about the implementation of special intervention strategies for early psychosis in your service what are your concerns? (Please be frank and use complete sentences.)

_____

_____

_____

_____

_____

_____

_____

_____

_____

_____

_____

Acknowledgements

This chapter is based on a paper presented at Hearing Voices: First International Conference on Qualitative Research in Early Intervention in Psychosis, which was held in Toronto on October 2007 (Rosen et al., 2007), and a poster presented at the International Conference in Early Intervention in Psychosis, which was held in Copenhagen on September 2002 (Gorrell et al., 2002). The author would like to thank the Commonwealth Department of Health and Aged Care for their financial assistance, all clinicians from Northern Sydney who were participating in this study, Beverley Moss for her participation in the related studies, Grainne Fadden for encouraging us to further develop this aspect of our study for publication, John Strauss, Sue Estroff, Katherine Boydell, and Sarah Bovaird for encouraging and supporting us through the preparation of this chapter, and Richard Nafa and Anne Streeter for their assistance in preparing this chapter.

References

Aarons, G.A. (2004). Mental health provider attitudes towards adoption of evidence-based practice: The Evidence-Based Practice Attitude Scale. *Mental Health Services Research, 6*(22), 61-74.

Anderson, T.B., and Forquer, S.L. (1982). Use of a concerns-based technical assistance model for quality assurance implementation. *Quality Review Bulletin, 8*(12), 4-11.

Brabban, A., and Kelly, M. (2008). A national survey of psychosocial intervention training and skills in early intervention services in England. *Journal of Mental Health Training, Education and Practice, 3*(2), 15–22.

Breitmayer, B.J., Ayres, L., and Knafi, K.A. (1993). Triangulation in qualitative research: Evaluation of completeness and confirmation purposes. *Journal of Nursing Scholarship, 25*(3), 237-43.

Callaly, T., and Arya, D. (2005). Leadership and management: Organizational change management in mental health. *Australian Psychiatry, 13*(2), 120-23.

Crocker, T., and Rissel, C. (1998). Knowledgè of, and attitudes to, the health outcomes approach among community mental health professionals. *Australian Health Review, 21*(4), 111-26.

Denzin, N.K. (1978). *Sociological methods.* New York: McGraw-Hill.

Denzin, N.K. (1989). *The Research Act* (3rd edition). New York: McGraw-Hill.

Fadden, G., and Palmer, M. (2008). Behavioural family therapy training for staff working in early intervention in psychosis. In G. Fadden (Ed.), *Meriden Family Intervention Newsletter for Early Intervention in Psychosis workers.* Birmingham, UK: Meriden West Midlands Mental Health Trusts.

Gavin, B., Cullen, W., Foley, S., McWilliams, S., Turner, N., O'Callaghan, E., and Bury, G. (2008). Integrating primary care and early intervention in psychosis services: A general practitioner perspective. *Early Intervention in Psychiatry*, *2*(2), 103-7.

Golop, R., Whitby, E., Buchanan, D., and Kentley, D. (2004). Influencing sceptical staff to become supporters of service improvement a qualitative study of doctors' and managers' views. *Quality and Safety in Health Care, 13*, 108-14.

Gorrell, J., Cornish, A., Nash, L., Miller, V., Tennant, C., and Rosen, A. (2002). *Clinician attitudes to early psychosis intervention* (paper presented at the International Conference on Early Intervention in Psychosis, Copenhagen, Denmark).

Gorrell, J., Cornish, A., Tennant, C., Rosen, A., Nash, L., McKay, D., and Moss, B. (2004a). Changes in early psychosis service provision: A file audit. *Australian and New Zealand Journal of Psychiatry, 38*, 687-93.

Gorrell, J., Moss, B., Ward, P.B., Nash, L., Tennant, C., Draganic, D., and Rosen, A. (2004b). *Pathways to care in early psychosis: Understanding treatment delay* (paper presented at the International Early Psychosis Conference, Vancouver, BC).

Gwele, N.S. (1996). Concerns of nurse educators regarding the implementation of a major curriculum reform. *Journal of Advanced Nursing, 24*(3), 607-14.

Hader, J.M., White, R., Lewis, S., Foreman, J.L., McDonald, P.W., Thompson, L.G. (2007). Doctors' views of clinical practice guidelines: A qualitative exploration using innovation theory. *Journal of Evaluation of Clinical Practice. 13*(4), 601-6.

Hall, G., George, A., and Rutherford, W. (1979). *Measuring stages of concern about the innovation: A manual for use of the SoC questionnaire*. Austin, TX: Research and Development Center for Teacher Education, University of Texas at Austin.

Hall, G.E., and Hord, S.M. (1987). *Change in schools*. Albany, NY: State University of New York Press.

Hall, G.E., Wallace, R.C., and Dossett, W.A. (1973). *A developmental conceptualization of the adoption process within educational institutions* (Report no. 3006). Austin, TX: Research and Development Center for Teacher Education, University of Texas at Austin.

Happell, B., Marti, T., and Pinikahana, J. (2003). Burnout and job satisfaction: A comparative study of psychiatric nurses from forensic and a mainstream mental health service. *International Journal of Mental Health Nursing, 12*(1), 39-47.

Harrison, M.E., McKay, M.M., and Bannon, W. (2004). Inner-city child mental health service use: The real question is why youth and families do not use services. *Community Mental Health Journal*, 40(2), 119-31.

Hodgins, G., Judd, F., Davis, J., and Faley, A. (2007). An integrated approach to general practice mental health training: The importance of context. *Australasian Psychiatry, 15*(1), 52-57.

Hord, S. (1987). *Evaluating Educational Innovation*. New York: Croon Helm.

Hord, S., Rutherford, W., Huling-Austin, L., and Hall, G. (1987). *Taking charge of change*. Alexandria, VA: Association for Supervision and Curriculum Development.

Jones, M., Bennett, J., Lucas, B., Miller, D., and Gray, R. (2007). Mental health nurse supplementary prescribing: Experiences of mental health nurses, psychiatrists and patients. *Journal of Advanced Nursing, 59*(5), 488-96.

Jordan-Marsh, M. (1985). Development of a tool for diagnosing changes in concern about exercise: A means of enhancing compliance. *Nursing Research, 34*(2), 103-7.

Kelly, M., O'Meara, H.A., and Smith J. (2007). Early intervention in psychosis: A rural perspective. *Journal of Psychiatric and Mental Health Nursing, 14*, 203-8.

Kimchi, J., Polivka, B., and Stevenson S.J. (1991). Triangulation: Operational definitions. *Nursing Research, 40*(6), 364-66.

Lewis, D. (1996). Computer-based patient education: Use by diabetes educators. *Diabetes Educator, 22*(2), 140-45.

Lewis, D., and Watson, J.E. (1997). Nursing faculty concerns regarding the adoption of computer technology. *Computers in Nursing, 15*(2), 71-76.

Magnusson, A., Hogberg, T., Lutzen, K., and Severinsson. E. (2004). Swedish mental health nurses' responsibility in supervised community care of persons with long-term mental illness. *Nursing and Health Sciences, 6*(1), 19-27.

McCann, T.V., Baird, J., Clark, E., and Lui, S. (2006). Beliefs about using consumer consultants in inpatient psychiatric units. *International Journal of Mental Health Nursing, 15*(4), 258-65.

McKay, D., Gorrell, J., Cornish, A., Tennant, C., Rosen, A., Moss, B., and Nash, L. (2006). Let's get physical: An audit of medical practice in first episode psychosis. *Australasian Psychiatry, 14*(2), 146-49.

McKinnon, D.H., and Nolan, P.C.J. (1989). Using computers in education: A concerns-based approach to professional development for teachers. *Australian Journal of Educational Technology, 5*(2), 113-31.

Miles, M.B., and Huberman, A.N. (1984). *Qualitative data analysis: A sourcebook of new methods.* Newbury Park, CA: Sage Publications.

Miller, V., Rosen, A., Parker, G.B., and Hartley, R. (1991). *A guide to standards of care and quality assurance for integrated mental health services.* Sydney, Australia: New South Wales Department of Health and University of NSW, Sydney.

Moss, B., and Gorrell, J. (2004). *A Tool to map the pathway to effective treatment for psychosis* (paper presented at the International Early Psychosis Conference, Vancouver, BC).

Nash. L., Gorrell, J., Cornish, A., Rosen, A., Miller, V., and Tennant, C. (2004) Clinical outcome of an early psychosis intervention program: Evaluation in a real-world context. *Australian and New Zealand Journal of Psychiatry, 38*, 694-701.

Newlove, B., and Hall, G. (1998). *A manual for assessing open-ended statements of concern about an innovation.* Austin, TX: Southwest Educational Laboratory.

Paxton, R., Chaplin, L., Selman, M., Liddon, A., Cramb, G., and Dodgson, G. (2003). Early intervention in psychosis: A pilot study of methods to help existing staff adapt. *Journal of Mental Health, 12*(6), 627-36.

Proudfoot, J., Jayasinghe, U.W., Holton, C., Grimm, J., Bubner, T., Amoroso, C., Harris, M.F. (2007). Team climate for innovation: What difference does it make in general practice? *International Journal for Quality in Health Care*, *19*(3), 164-69.

Rogers, E.M. (1983). *The diffusion of innovation* (3rd edition). New York: Free Press.

Rosen, A., Gorrell, J., Cornish, A., Miller, V., Tennant, C., Nash, L., Moss, B., McKay, D. (2007). *Clinician attitudes towards early psychosis intervention: Triangulation of method and stages of concern—Northern Sydney Health Early Psychosis Project* (invited presentation to first Conference on Qualitative Research in Early Intervention in Psychosis, Hospital for Sick Children, Toronto).

Senge, P.M. (1990). *The fifth discipline: The art and practice of the learning organization*. New York: Doubleday Currency.

Van Dorn, R.A., Swartz, M.S., Elbogen, E.B., Swanson, J.W., Kim, M., Ferron, J., McDaniel, L.A., and Scheyett, A.M. (2006). Clinicians' attitudes regarding barriers to the implementation of psychiatric advance directives. *Administration and Policy in Mental Health and Mental Health Services Research*, *33*(4), 449-60.

7

Ironic Interventions: Balancing Risks and Rewards in First Episode Psychosis via Qualitative Inquiry

Sue E. Estroff

In this agnostic reflection on interventions for first episode and early psychosis, I consider whether and how qualitative inquiry can inform and influence clinical and research approaches to early intervention in psychosis. As with other treatments such as chemotherapy and major surgery, interventions for psychosis, early and late, frequently require further interventions (not always effective) to counteract their consequences. What is especially ironic in this case is that early intervention is meant to avoid, reduce, and otherwise derail the "psychosocial toxicity" of "self-imposed stigma, restrictions on life goals and needless fear in response to false labelling" associated with treatment (McGorry and Warner, 2002, p. 543; Warner, 2003).[1]

The desirability of treatments designed specifically for people in the early phases of psychosis is not in dispute. Emerging findings from both descriptive and controlled trial research are encouraging and also in the early stages of refinement and replication (Addington et al., 2007; Marshall and Rathbone, 2006). It is beyond the scope of this chapter to reprise the energetic and entirely necessary debate about the underlying assumptions, risks, and rewards as well as the adequacy of the evidence for early intervention (McGorry, 2008; Pelosi, 2008; Salonkangas and McGlashan, 2008; Warner, 2003). However, in view of many indicators that treatment itself can be debilitating, physically and psychically, we have a heightened interest in reducing, if not eliminating, noxious by-products of receiving care (for example, Birchwood, 2003; McCay et al., 2006; Neugeboren, 1997). As a result, we cast a skeptical and hopeful gaze on how research using qualitative methods can provide evidence of the risks and rewards of interventions for people whose experiences with psychosis and treatment are emergent, recent, and unfamiliar. My concerns are with an analysis and critique of the underlying paradigms, language promises, treatment modalities, risks, and potential (yet predictable) welcome and unwelcome outcomes of early intervention and first episode interventions.

There is considerable agreement that the most sought after, and probably elusive, outcome for people with first episode psychosis (FEP) is that they may lead rich, active, and meaningful lives, unyoked from the fear, shame, and discrimination attributable to their illness or treatment (Bonney and Stickley, 2008). There is a similar consensus that the experiences of onset, identification, and treatment of early psychosis are frequently traumatic and life altering for the person and often for their families and loved ones (Birchwood, 2003; MacInnes and Lewis, 2008; McCay et al., 2006). To illustrate, the Camden and Islington Early Intervention Service (2009) state: "The main aims of the service include to maximise both symptomatic and social recovery after a first episode of psychosis; and to make first experiences of service contact less aversive and stigmatising from service users' perspectives."

We know a great deal from first-person narratives, psychiatric consumer activism, and qualitative research about "symptoms of treatment" as well as recovery (Crossley and Crossley, 2001; Davidson, Schmutte, Dinzeo, and Andres-Hyman, 2008; Estroff, 2004; Hopper, 2007). Symptoms of treatment refer to the demeaning, damaging, and otherwise anti-therapeutic effects of various aspects of treatment—including medication side effects, forced treatment, effects of corrosive interactions with clinicians on self-concept and identity, self-esteem, and well-being, and the erosion of sociality and meaningful lives due to self-and-other stigma and discrimination (Deegan, 1993). A warning sounded by David Granger (1994, p. 3) is concise and chilling: "Don't let your treatment interfere with your recovery."

The widespread embrace of "recovery" language and practices in many quarters derives in part from the persuasive force of consumer and family members' critiques of what treatment has been provided and how. Comparable inquiry among early intervention and first episode participants is in the early stages (Boydell and others in this volume; Judge, Estroff, Perkins, and Penn, 2008). It is worth examining why there is vibrant international psychiatric adult consumer activism, often in response to current treatment practices and policies. We are engaged in expanding the reach of interventions to more and younger patients within a preventive framework. It is reasonable to include identifying and reducing offending practices and policies as important goals of care. This is a broad area of investigation well suited for consumer–researcher collaborative work using an array of methods.

The Promise (and Peril) of Qualitative Research

Both the study of, and study in, early intervention and first episode treatment deserve the attention of scholars from various backgrounds.[2] The use of inductive approaches to explore emergent and complicated topics can be combined with clinical and health services survey data collection and analysis or may stand alone. Social and behavioural scientists as well as scholars in the humanities, and increasingly in medicine, take varying approaches to qualitative work, but they have in common a focus on developing what Clifford Geertz (1973) refers to as "thick description"—an accounting of words, meanings, sensations, actions, and symbols that illuminates but does not necessarily simplify. Inductive methods of inquiry may be particularly powerful in search of unanticipated phenomena and deeply felt but difficult to communicate experiences. The eclectic repertoire of systematic data collection, combined with analytic rigor, can complicate and enrich knowledge rather than standardize or reduce it.

Study In

In the case of FEP, a rationale for qualitative inquiry might be expressed as follows:

- There are gaps in knowledge and evidence of how people recognize, respond to, and make sense of psychosis in the early stages and how engagement in treatment affects personal and social identity, sensate experience and bodily habitat, internalized and external stigma, and emerging concepts of personhood.
- Qualitative methods are designed to retrieve authenticities of experience—the subjectivities of patients, families, and clinicians—in their own terms and modes of expression.
- An informed understanding of subjective experiences of psychosis and treatment is essential to preserving and enhancing the personhood of people in the first and early stages.
- Incorporating these findings into treatment paradigms and interventions could lead to better outcomes for patients, particularly those associated with personhood and lives of meaning and opportunity.

This formulation is, of course, speculative and optimistic and focuses on the participants and recipients of interventions. The authors in this volume illustrate some of the earliest qualitative research in these areas, and the results make clear that the work is imaginative, feasible, and illuminating. Whether and how this ongoing and future inquiry will inform, and be incorporated into, first episode research and interventions remains to be seen.

Study Of

The other significant warrant for qualitative analysis and critique concerns the field and practice of early intervention itself. As a "movement" with a variety of intellectual, ethical, social policy, pharmaceutical, and advocacy constituencies, the entire research and intervention enterprise deserves attention (Pelosi, 2008). There has already been a remarkable period of discussion and debate about the protocols and practices for research and intervention (McGorry, 2008; McGorry and Warner, 2002; Pelosi, 2008). This emerging articulation of concepts, evidence, risk benefit (moral, clinical, and financial), inclusion in research protocols, work force issues, and how key variables are defined is ripe for archival and ethnographic inquiry and analysis.

Objects and Subjects of Interest: Of and In

Vocabularies and Concepts

In a provocative essay entitled "Preventing Chronic Disease: The Dark Side of a Bright Idea," Deborah Stone (1990) outlines some concerns we should have about the vocabulary of early intervention in psychosis. She suggests the need for "a professional self-awareness about the moral assumptions and political context of risk-factor theory." Health researchers do not simply "reveal" pure relationships between the hazards and health that exist in nature. Rather as they create a body of knowledge that constitutes our societal understanding of disease etiology, they structure our views of causality, our moral choices about where to attribute blame for the disease, and our policy choices about how to allocate the material burdens" (ibid., p. 99). Stone points out that the application of at-risk categories can contribute to reducing access to insurance, employment, and other life opportunities. Of particular relevance in the early intervention in psychosis area are the following concepts and vocabularies.

Risk: At, High, Very High, and Elevated for Developing Psychosis or Converting

While there is progress towards developing empirically sound criteria for various kinds of risk, even the most optimistic advocates agree that false positive rates are between 50 and 60 percent (McGorry, 2008). In fact, the 2002 statement of consensus on early intervention in schizophrenia precludes early interventions with asymptomatic or sub-threshold persons given the current state of knowledge and the potential harms of antipsychotic medication (McGorry and Warner, 2003). Still, the vocabulary of risk remains central to the research enterprise and would benefit from ongoing examination—both in the published literature and in clinical settings. This work would best be accomplished in a collaborative setting among clinician researchers and scholars from both socio-medical and humanities perspectives. A multidisciplinary group would be less likely to privilege assumptions or findings from a single perspective and would perhaps engender reciprocal reflexive analysis among all of the investigators.

Prodromal, Pre-Psychotic, Sub-Threshold

The definition and identification of these categories is susceptible to significant variability and malleability. Taken to an extreme, the prodrome or pre-psychotic period could characterize an individual's entire life—up to the point of developing psychotic symptoms. How and when the temporal window of the prodomal period is decided upon by researchers will be of considerable interest. Here we encounter a re-writing of the patient's biography from a clinical point of view. Qualitative inquiry with clinicians, patients, and families could contribute other versions of events and experiences—a narrative presence for autobiography and second-person narratives in our understanding of the natural history of psychosis.

Duration of Untreated Psychosis

Not only is there controversy about the importance of this concept in prognosis but also in determining when to start the clock (Warner, 2003). What is at stake is whether there are sufficient grounds for increasingly earlier intervention. The allure of prevention is understandably strong when psychosis may be looming. What mechanisms within and outside the field will moderate and mediate the desire to halt, slow, or derail such a dreaded outcome.

Burden and Cost

One of the ways that researchers and advocates seek resources for, and attention to, their particular interests is to estimate and then publicize the burdens (on society and families) and costs (of treatment and lost productivity). While these may be effective strategies at some level, they can also unintentionally exaggerate public concern about the drain on resources and impel policy makers to draconian measures to control costs. We should carefully monitor the deployment of cost and burden language in the early intervention area as well as the results.

Underlying Assumptions

Along with, and clearly related to, concepts and terminologies are the underlying assumptions, theories, and models upon which experimentation and innovation rest. Raimo Salonkangas and Thomas McGlashan

(2008) describe two primary models for early intervention in psychosis: vulnerability and a hybrid of various patterns and processes. Yet, underlying these and other theories is the "early is better" assumption. As they explain it, "if we can prevent schizophrenia in its very early phase or before the occurrence of its psychotic stage, or even if we can shorten the duration of untreated psychosis, we can protect the individual from severe suffering and from clinical and psychosocial consequences" (ibid., p. 93). Richard Warner (2003) provides a convincing historical account of this idea, which has underlaid much of psychiatry for a very long time. At a recent gathering of the National Institute of Mental Health (NIMH) study section members, Thomas Insel, director of the NIMH, described psychosis as "the end stage of the disease of schizophrenia," comparable to a stroke or heart attack being the end stage of cardiovascular disease (personal communication, 9 June 2008). Thus, we should screen for, attempt to prevent, and eventually eliminate this disease as we would cancer or heart disease. With this model, we have the opportunity to examine the gains and challenges of an aggressive preventive regime that is thoroughly medicalized.

Prior to its current re-embrace among schizophrenia researchers, the vulnerability model had, and still retains, tremendous appeal and application in social and behaviour sciences, particularly in combination with studies of social stress and morbidity. As Frank Furedi (2004, p. 414) notes, "vulnerability has become a key concept of our times. We talk about vulnerable people, vulnerable communities, vulnerable women, vulnerable children... Indeed we use the term so frequently that we know longer have to ask 'vulnerable to what'? For the only possible answer to this question is 'vulnerability to everything.'" The researchable question at hand is how the vulnerability notion is adopted by the public, by patients and their families, and by researchers and with what results. Furedi argues that the contemporary "vulnerable self" undermines subjectivity and human agency, disempowering people and suggesting that they must be vigilant to self-protect or to seek professional help to counter their shortcomings. On the other hand, one could argue that the vulnerability model is more multi-dimensional and less passivity-inducing than an orthodox medical, disease-based formulation.

Preserving Personhood: Outcomes, Labelling, Insight, Denial, and Medication

Perhaps the most important areas for qualitative work in early intervention revolve around the preservation of personhood, of the subjective sense of self as worthy, recognizable, and purposeful. Elizabeth McCay et al. (2006) and D.L. MacInnes and M. Lewis (2008) report some of the earliest systematic attention to this constellation of concerns in first episode interventions. There is also resonant and relevant work under the guise of recovery (Bonney and Stickley, 2008; Davidson, Schmutte, Dinzeo, and Andres-Hyman, 2008; Hopper, 2007). At issue is how the participants in treatment programs experience not only the interventions but also themselves and not only while they are in treatment but also for years later (Ritscher and Phelan, 2004). What we describe as "outcomes" are, from another perspective, their lives. Max Marshall and John Rathbone (2006, p. 21) surmise that in the studies they reviewed, "no improvements in quality of life occurred in the early intervention group, even though they were given cognitive behavioural therapy. However, they also received risperidone which may have negated any gains in quality of life, due to its adverse effects profile." What we describe as good outcomes in symptom reduction may not translate into good outcomes in other domains that are as, if not more, important to the participants. Maria Mattson, Alain Topor, Johan Culberg, and Yvonne Forsell (2008) report that the people they considered to be "recovered" five years after first episode treatment had fewer financial resources (financial strain) and smaller, less affectively engaged social networks than the control group. What we describe as a lack of insight and denial of illness may be something else altogether—attempts at self-preservation, at biographical coherence, and as resistance to a stigmatized or spoiled identity. Would we consider a life lived in fear of recurrence of psychosis, and thus adherence to medication, a good outcome? Alternately, vigilant self-management of symptoms and life routines that reduce stress and maintain well-being might result from effective first episode treatment that gives the person hope for recovery. In view of the serious risks of first-line antipsychotic medication that is predominant in early intervention, are we investigating with equal intensity other forms of treatment? All of these areas of inquiry are especially well suited to longitudinal, depth, multi-method, qualitative investigation. Katherine Boydell and her colleagues in this volume have demonstrated with remarkable clarity the power of research methods, analysis, and representation that go beyond text and scales.

Skepticism and Promise for Future Inquiry

At this juncture, the promise and potential of qualitative inquiry in this fascinating domain are alluring yet unrealized. Yet there are cautions for us as well. Can we avoid colonizing the biographies of research participants with clinical, cultural, and narrative tropes? Can the research enterprise itself be therapeutic, expressive, and subjectively enhancing for our subjects? Or will this kind of research relationship be stressful and unsettling? How will we respond to subjects who may disagree with our representations of them? Is this an inherently exploitative enterprise on our part?

Our tasks include providing persuasive data and findings so that clinical enthusiasm and research are informed by findings with lives lived in "the real world." Prevention is a compelling, common-sense, and potent enterprise. However, it is important to remember Clifton Meador's (1994, p. 441) article "The Last Well Person," which he concludes: "In my imagined meeting with the last well person I can hear myself saying, 'Doing all those boring things you do to stay healthy may or may not make you live longer. However, I am sure of one thing; it will make your life seem longer."

Notes

1 McGorry and Warner (2002) use the term "psychosocial toxicity" to describe the potential effects of untreated psychosis. I use it here to characterize the opposite, the effects of treatment.

2 Here I am harkening back to Elliott Freidson's (1961) distinction of sociology *in* medicine (patients' experiences and symptoms, responses to illness, outcomes, access to care, and so on) and sociology *of* medicine (medical practices and culture, ethics, how evidence is gathered and construed, and how interventions are developed and deployed).

References

Addington, J., Cadenhead, K.S., Cannon, T.D., Cornblatt, B., McGlashan, T.H., Perkins, D.O., and Heinssen, R. (2007). North American Prodrome Longitudinal Study: A collaborative multisite approach to prodromal schizophrenia research. *Schizophrenia Bulletin, 33*(3), 665-72.

Birchwood, M. (2003). Pathways to emotional dysfunction in first episode psychosis. *British Journal of Psychiatry, 18*, 373-75.

Bonney, S., and Stickley, T. (2008). Recovery and mental health: A review of the British literature. *Journal of Psychiatric and Mental Health Nursing, 15*, 140-53.

Camden and Islington Early Intervention Service. (2009). International Early Psychosis Association. Online: http://www.iepa.org.

Crossley, M.L, and Crossley, N. (2001). "Patient" voices, social movements and the habitus: How psychiatric survivors "speak out." *Social Science and Medicine, 52*, 1477-89.

Davidson, L., Schmutte, T., Dinzeo, T., and Andres-Hyman, R. (2008). Remission and recovery in schizophrenia: Practitioner and patient perspectives. *Schizophrenia Bulletin, 34*(1), 5-8.

Deegan, P.E. (1993). Recovering our sense of value after being labeled mentally ill. *Journal of Psychosocial Nursing and Mental Health Services, 31*(4), 7-11.

Estroff, S.E. (2004). Subject/subjectivities in dispute: The politics and poetics of first person narratives of schizophrenia. In R. Barrett and J. Jenkins (Eds.), *The edge of experience: Schizophrenia, culture, and subjectivity* (pp. 282-302). Cambridge: Cambridge University Press.

Freidson, E. (1961). The sociology of medicine. *Current Sociology, 10*: 123-40.

Furedi, F. (2004). Reflections on the medicalisation of social experience. *British Journal of Guidance and Counselling, 32*(3), 413-15.

Geertz, C. (1973). Thick description. In C. Geertz, *The interpretation of cultures* (pp. 3-33). New York: Basic Books.

Granger, D. (1994). Recovery from Mental Illness: A First Person Perspective of an Emerging Paradigm. Presented at the First National Conference on Recovery from Mental Illness. Columbus, Ohio. April 1994 [unpublished].

Hopper, K. (2007). Rethinking social recovery in schizophrenia: What a capabilities approach might offer. *Social Science and Medicine, 65*, 868-79.

Judge, A., Estroff, S., Perkins, D.O., and Penn, D.L. (2008). Recognizing and responding to early psychosis: A qualitative analysis of individual narratives. *Psychiatric Services, 59*, 96-99.

MacInnes, D.L., and Lewis, M. (2008). The evaluation of a short group programme to reduce self stigma in people with serious and enduring mental health problems. *Journal of Psychiatric and Mental Health Nursing, 15*, 59-65.

Marshall, M., and Rathbone, J. (2006). Early intervention for psychosis. *Cochrane Database of Systematic Reviews, 28*(3), 1-75.

Mattsson, M., Topor, A., Cullberg, J., and Forsell, Y. (2008). Association between financial strain, social network and five-year recovery from first episode psychosis. *Social Psychiatry and Psychiatric Epidemiology, 43*(12), 947-52.

McCay, E., Beanlands, H., Leszcz, M., Goering, P., Ryan, K., Seeman, M.V., Vishevsky, T. (2006). A group intervention to promote healthy self-concepts and guide recovery in first episode schizophrenia: A pilot study. *Psychiatric Rehabilitation Journal, 30*, 105-11.

McGorry, P.D. (2008.) Is early intervention in the major psychiatric disorders justified? Yes. *British Medical Journal, 695*, 337-38.

McGorry, P.D., and Warner, R. (2002). Consensus on early intervention in schizophrenia. *Schizophrenia Bulletin, 28*(3), 543-44.

Meador, C.K. (1994). The last well person. *New England Journal of Medicine, 330*(6), 440-41.

Neugeboren, J. (1997). *Imagining Robert.* New York: Morrow.

Pelosi, A. (2008). Is early intervention in the major psychiatric disorders justified? No. *British Medical Journal, 710*, 337-38.

Ritsher, J.B., and Phelan, J.C. (2004). Internalized stigma predicts erosion of morale among psychiatric outpatients. *Psychiatry Research, 129*, 257-65.

Salonkangas, R.K.R., and McGlashan T.H. (2008). Early detection and intervention of psychosis: A review. *Nordic Journal of Psychiatry, 62*(2), 92-105.

Stone, D. (1990). Preventing chronic disease: The dark side of a bright idea. In Institute of Medicine of the National Academies (Ed.), *Chronic disease and disability: Beyond the acute medical model.* Washington, DC: Institute of Medicine of the National Academies.

Warner, R. (2003). Fact versus fantasy: A reply to Bentall and Morrison. *Journal of Mental Health, 12*(4), 351-57.

Conclusion

Katherine M. Boydell, H. Bruce Ferguson, and Sarah J. Bovaird

Mental health interventions are increasingly complex (Larsen, 2007), involving a number of different "active ingredients" to achieve change (Medical Research Council, 2000). Understanding the contexts and ways in which such interventions achieve their effects is crucial for scientific understanding and effective clinical delivery (Campbell et al., 2000). The "phased" development of complex interventions has been advocated (Medical Research Council, 2000), and there is interest in the role of qualitative methods alongside randomized controlled trials (Lewin, Glenton and Oxman, 2009). Qualitative research can help to explore some of this complexity and increase our understanding of the subjective experience of those impacted by psychosis and the ways in which interventions are used and experienced (Khan, Bower, and Rogers, 2007).

This book has featured a series of qualitative research studies in the area of early psychosis that contribute to our understanding of the complex, little-understood personal, interpersonal, and social processes experienced by individuals who have experienced first episode psychosis (FEP). They demonstrate the need for the active engagement of the individual suffering from psychosis in making sense of his or her experience and suggest that individuals should be understood from within their own framework of meaning. These studies offer much needed data on the factors, other than routine treatment and early interventions, which are most likely to make a difference in the lives of youth with early psychosis and those who care for and support them. Specifically, the subjective experience of youth, their families, and service providers have been highlighted; the importance of attending to the individualized nature of each person's explanations and beliefs around their experience of psychosis, shaped in part by their own particular cultural and social context. Embracing young people's individual meaning and attributions for psychosis cultivates effective techniques for treatment and the sustainment of hope. The qualitative research methods that are employed in these studies have the potential to effectively capture the significance of meaning making that permeates the experiences of young people who have suffered from a first episode of psychosis, the families that support them, and the caregivers who work with them.

Hearing the "voice" of families and caregivers allows for the development of practical ways to support them and involve them in interventions when doing so is appropriate. Examining the response of professionals to interacting with, and treating, young people during an FEP facilitates the evolution of training for effective and sustained intervention and assists us in modifying our systems to provide more accessible and appropriate care. Qualitative inquiry has a critical role in future work regarding what constitutes elements of effective services and supports and, thus, in helping us understand the role of implementation science and its impact on changing attitudes and behaviour.

The contexts and ways in which early intervention programs are used and experienced have also been underscored. Although the studies that are reviewed make an important contribution to our understanding of the lived experience of psychosis as well as providing richly textured accounts of the social context in which psychosis is identified and treated, much work remains. Currently, the weight of published qualitative research falls within the realm of the subjective experience of psychosis and help seeking. This focus reflects the early intervention field's emphasis on reducing the duration of untreated psychosis (DUP). However, as this area advances, more qualitative research is required to address treatment and recovery, namely intervention practices, social relationships, and education and work activities. In particular, the school as an important social setting for young people has been neglected. In addition, few qualitative studies elicit the subjective experience of school personnel, friends, siblings, and others who play important roles in the life of a young person experiencing psychosis.

Despite the increasing number of qualitative studies conducted in the health sciences, these investigations largely remain isolated works as few attempts are made to draw inferences from similar or related studies (Estabrooks, Field, and Morse, 1994). As such, results from qualitative projects continue to be obscured, and this occurrence reduces their potential impact on clinical practice, research, and health policy. Carole Estabrooks, Peggy Anne Field, and Janice Morse (1994, p. 503) note that the analysis and synthesis of findings from a number of qualitative studies may "increase the level of abstraction, lead to greater generalizability, and...can lead to the development of mid-range theory." When the findings of several studies are synthesized, more emphasis is placed on theorizing and recontextualizing as patterns emerge from the findings, resulting in a contribution to the construction of theory that is more powerful than any single study" (p. 505). Although the synthesis of research is important in theory development and at the pragmatic level in knowledge transfer between academia and decision-making audiences, there is a need to move beyond this synthesis and to engage in conversations, collaborations, and a reinterpretation of the research evidence in innovative ways in order for knowledge to be more usable and specific to particular contexts (Pope, Mays, and Popay, 2006). Indeed, the initial responses of audiences to interpretive works such as the dance production profiled in Chapter 2 of this volume suggest that such knowledge translation initiatives may provide unexpected channels for communication of research results and stigma reduction (Boydell and Jackson, 2010).

There is a dearth of qualitative longitudinal studies in FEP (Boydell, Staiuslis, Volpe, and Gladstone, 2010). Longitudinal research would focus on the unfolding of process in time and move beyond "contextualized snapshots of processes and people," allowing for an examination of changes that occur in the lives of young people over time and the processes associated with these changes (Farrell, 1996, p. 10).

Qualitative inquiry in the field of early intervention, more often than not, renders the lived experience of participants as communicated by the researcher as unproblematic—thus, future inquiry would benefit from a more critical examination of the epistemological and ideological assumptions that underlie the particular methods used. Sue Estroff in Chapter 7 in this volume cautions us regarding the potential perils of engaging in this work. An emphasis on reflexivity—systematically attending to the knowledge and awareness of the researcher's contribution to the construction of meanings throughout the research process—would contribute to transparency in the process of qualitative inquiry (Mruck and Breuer, 2003).

Substantively, through the use of qualitative methods, the richness of human experience and the "voice of the other" are profiled (Jones, 2004, p. 97). The subjective meaning constructions of people with psychosis and other key stakeholders in early psychosis constitute an important source of knowledge and a potential contribution to our understandings of the recognition, definition, and legitimization of a problem, the pathway to care, treatment services and supports attained, and the process of recovery. There remain many unsolved issues and questions surrounding FEP. These will demand the continued use of qualitative studies to provide insights to improving early identification and service delivery. Primary among these unresolved questions is the aspiration of reducing the DUP. Qualitative studies are needed to continue to map the lived experience of youth, their families, and others in their social network as the best strategy for reducing the DUP. It is critical to point out here that the essential ingredients in effective early intervention that still need to be studied are not only mental health in nature but also include the important role of the school, work, and peer support networks.

The concept for this book was born out of an international symposium hosted in Toronto, Ontario, in October 2007, which was focused on collaborative research as a systemic way to change front-line practice. The symposium brought together leading international researchers to highlight qualitative research that reveals the voice of young people affected by psychosis, their families, and the practitioners who serve them. Both the symposium and this book are examples of collaborative work and highlight the importance of examining different perspectives from the micro to the macro level as well as caveats to continually examine the assumptions and consequences of our work. As the field continues to move forward, it is important to remember the importance of collaborative work with a broad range of stakeholders including young people experiencing psychosis and their families. FEP is a complex disorder, which evolves slowly in the multiple dimensions of daily life. If we are to understand the disorder and intervene effectively with interventions that will by necessity continue to be complex, then we will have to continue with research strategies that bring us all together in this work. This book, and our work, is dedicated to this cause.

References

Boydell, K.M., Stasiulis, E., Volpe, T., and Gladstone, B. (2010). A descriptive review of qualitative studies in first episode psychosis. *Early Intervention in Psychiatry, 4,* 7-24. doi: 10.1111/j.1751-7893.2009.00154.x.

Boydell, K.M., and Jackson, S. (2010). *Research-based dance as knowledge translation strategy.* Ottawa, ON: Canadian Institutes for Health Research.

Campbell, M., Fitzpatrick, R., Haines, A., Kinmonth, A.L, Sandercock, P., Spiegelhalter, D., and Tyrer, P. (2000). Framework for design and evaluation of complex interventions to improve health. *British Medical Journal, 321,* 694-96.

Estabrooks, C.A., Field, P.A., and Morse, J.M. (1994). Aggregating qualitative findings: An approach to theory development. *Qualitative Health Research, 4,* 503-11.

Farrell, S. (1996). *What is qualitative longitudinal research?* London: London School of Economics and Political Sciences Methodology Institute.

Jones, K. (2004). Mission drift in qualitative research, or moving toward a systematic review of qualitative studies, moving back to a more systemic narrative review. *Qualitative Report, 9*(1), 95-112.

Khan, N., Bower, P., and Rogers, A. (2007). Guided self-help in primary care mental health: Meta-synthesis of qualitative studies of patient experience. *British Journal of Psychiatry,* 191, 206-11.

Larsen, J. (2007). Understanding a complex intervention: Person-centred ethnography in early psychosis. *Journal of Mental Health,* 16(3), 333-445.

Lewin, S., Glenton, C., and Oxman, A.D. (2009). Use of qualitative methods alongside randomised controlled trials of complex healthcare interventions: Methodological study. *British Medical Journal,* 339(3496), 1-7.

Medical Research Council. (2000). *A framework for development and evaluation of RCTs for complex interventions to improve health.* London: Medical Research Council.

Mruck, K., and Breuer, F. (2003). Subjectivity and reflexivity in qualitative research: The FQS issues. *Forum: Qualitative Social Research,* 4(2), Article 23. Online: http://nbn-resolving.de/urn:nbn:de:0114-fqs0302233.

Pope, C., Mays, C., and Popay, J. (2006). Informing policy making and management in health care: The place for synthesis. *Healthcare Policy,* 1(2), 43-48.

Index

Titles in the SickKids Community and Mental Health Series
Published by Wilfrid Laurier University Press

Hearing Voices: Qualitative Inquiry in Early Psychosis, edited by
Katherine M. Boydell and H. Bruce Ferguson 2012 / 156 pp. /
ISBN 978-1-55458-263-1

Preventing Eating-Related and Wei   *Disorder Collaborative
Research, Advocacy, and Policy C*   McVey, Michael
P. Levine, Nina Piran, and I   ing 2012 /
ISBN 978-1-55458-340-9

Youth, Education, a   *.s*, edited
by Kate Tilliczek an   /
ISBN 978-1-55458-634-

*Understanding and Addressing Girls' Aggressive Behaviour: A Focus on
Relationships*, edited by Debra J. Pepler and H. Bruce Ferguson / forth-
coming 2013 / ISBN 978-1-55458-838-1